Review on Amazon

Scan me

Make • Color • Commit™

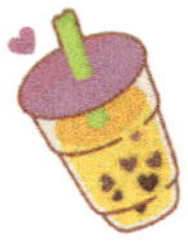

- The images and recipes in this book are NOT AI generated. These recipes are created by real creators for real people.

  Visit our website for details:

  www. smoothiequeen.blog

- Replace two meals a day with our recommended Smoothie recipes in this book. Don't worry, if you ever feel lost, check out our website where daily recipes are posted real creators

- After making your Smoothie, color away how your drink looks like and then enjoy it. This keeps you focused in a fun way.

- Not only will you rejuvenate your mind and body over a course of 30 days, you will shed some body fat also. (Individual results may vary)

Disclaimer:
The recipes in this book are provided for educational and inspirational purposes only. They are not intended as medical advice. Before starting any new diet or nutrition plan – especially one that replaces meals – consult your physician or a qualified healthcare provider to ensure it's right for your individual needs.

Introduction - Why This 30-Day Reset Works

This 30-day plan is not a strict diet or a quick fix — it's a gentle reset for your digestion, energy, and overall wellbeing. By using smoothies and high-protein meals in a smart, structured way, you give your body a break from overload while still getting the nutrients it needs.

Each phase is designed to support your stomach, reduce inflammation, and improve how you feel — physically and emotionally. No calorie counting. No extreme restrictions. Just a simple rhythm your body can trust.

You'll go step by step:

Week 1 - full smoothie days with protein at night,

Week 2 - spaced smoothies and light rhythm,

Week 3 - hearty mornings, smoothies later,

Week 4 - protein at midday, light start and end.

By Day 30, your body will not only feel lighter — it will function better.

Let's begin.

Day 1 – Relief

Smoothies replace breakfast and lunch, protein-rich dinner.

Sunrise Pink Smoothie:

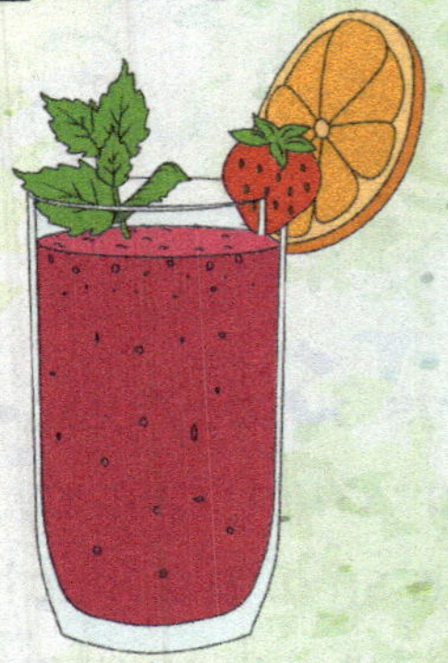

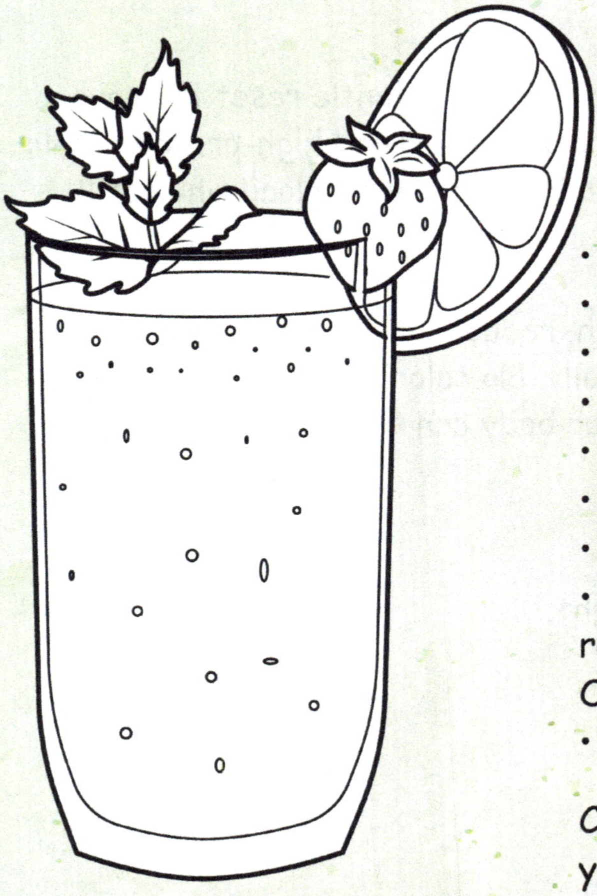

- Orange: 1 medium (peeled)
- Carrot: 1 medium (chopped, ~1/2 cup)
- Small beetroot: 1 (chopped, ~1/2 cup)
- Frozen strawberries: 1 cup
- Frozen zucchini: 0.5 cup
- Frozen raspberries: 1 cup
- Roasted cashews: 0.5 cup
- Plant-based milk: 1.5 cups (coconut milk recommended)

Optional Sweeteners:

- 1 small banana or 2 pitted Medjool dates

Calories~200-250 per serving (varies with milk, yogurt type, and added sweeteners).

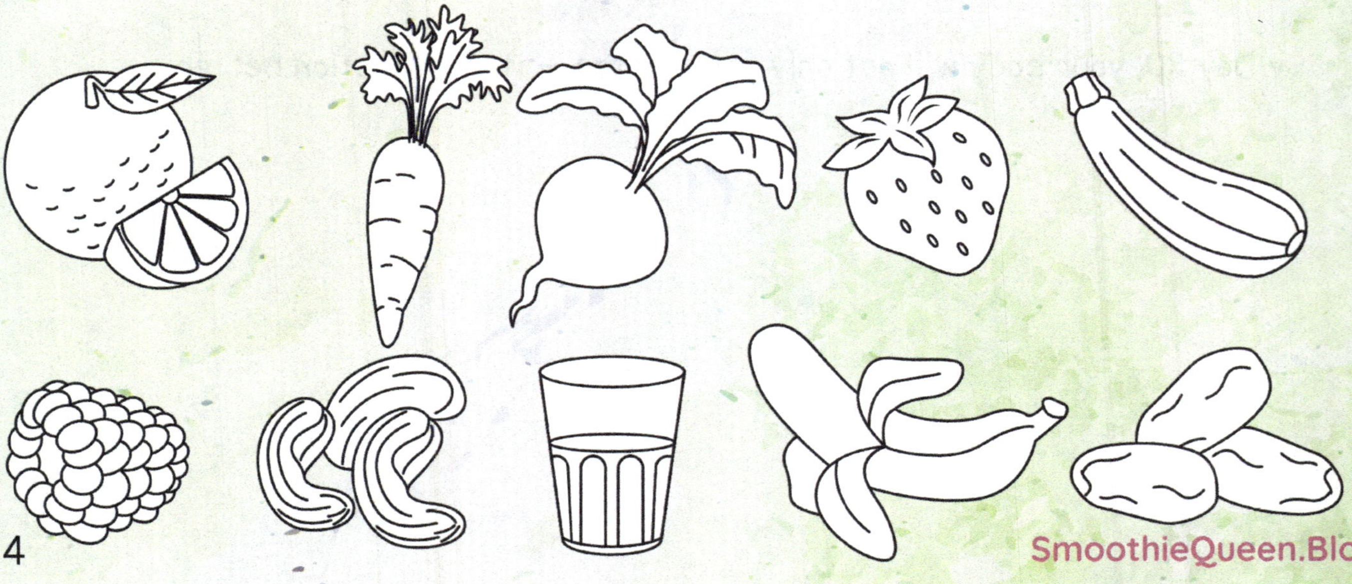

Bloating and heaviness begin to fade. A protein-rich dinner keeps you full without overloading the digestive system.

Green Detox Smoothie:

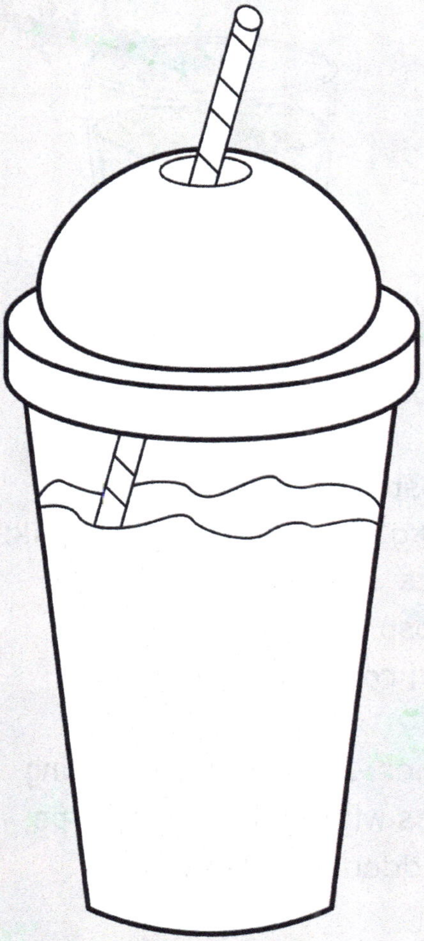

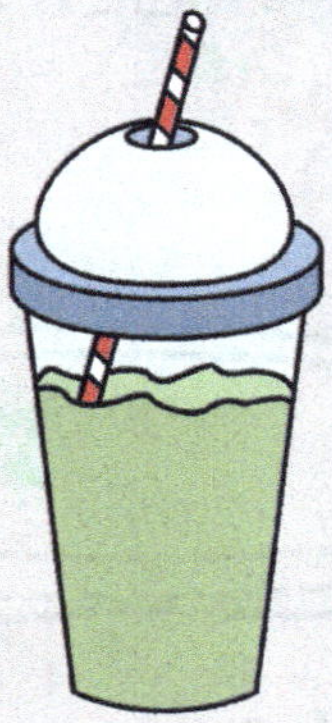

•1 cup lettuce leaves (butter lettuce or romaine work best)
•¼ cup fresh mint leaves
1 medium avocado, pitted and peeled
•½ cup coconut milk (canned or carton)
•1–2 tsp erythritol (or stevia to taste)
•1 tbsp lemon juice
•½ cup water (adjust for desired thickness)
Optional: Pinch of sea salt or a handful of spinach for extra greens

Calories~200-250 per serving (varies with milk, yogurt type, and added sweeteners).

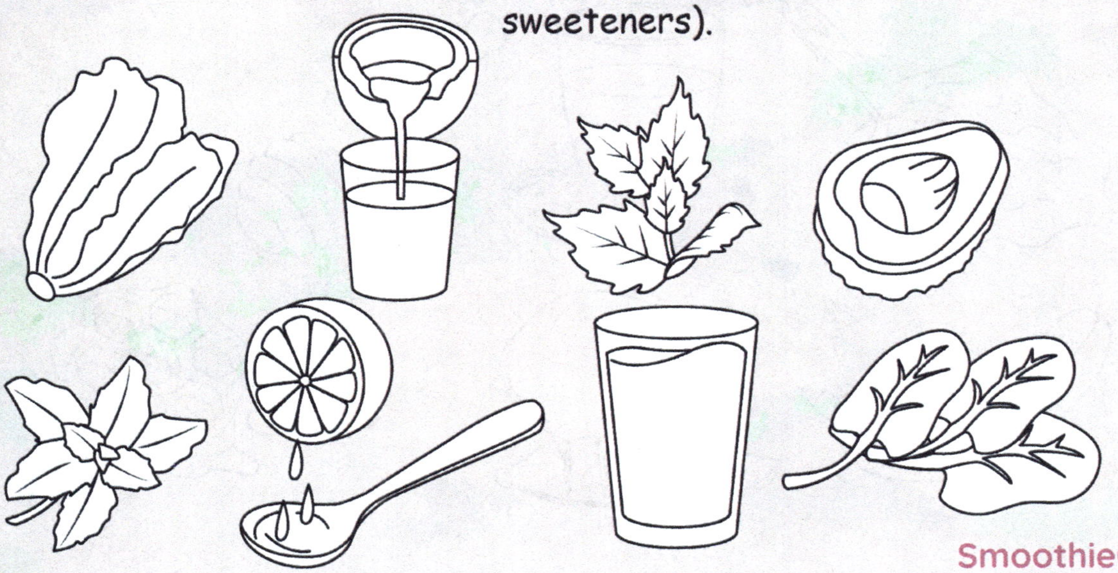

Day 2 – Gentle Detox Begins

Smoothies replace breakfast and lunch, protein-rich dinner.

Matcha Green Tea:

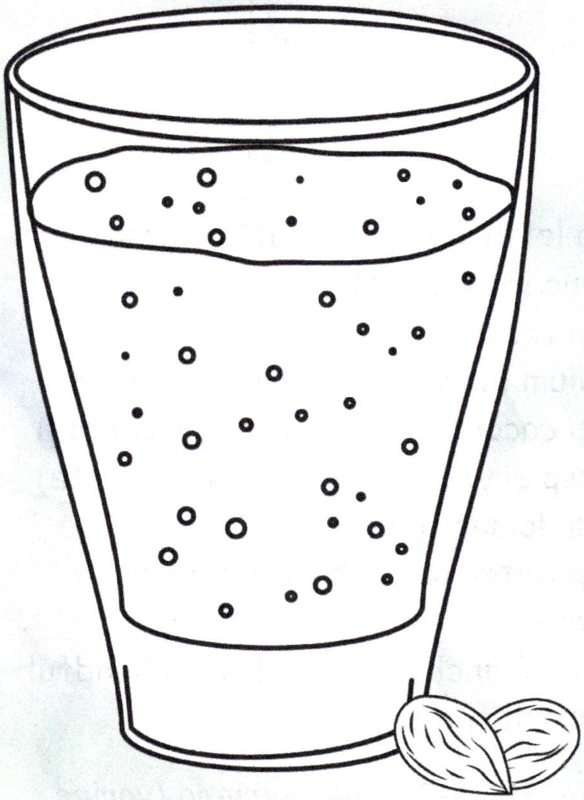

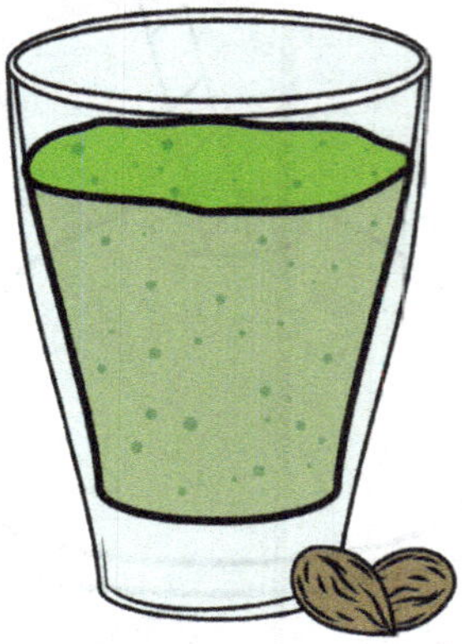

- 1 tbsp. Matcha powder,
- 300 g almond or coconut milk;
- 2 pcs. bananas;
- 2 tbsp. honey;
- 1/2 Frozen mango

Calories~200-250 per serving (varies with milk, yogurt type, and added sweeteners).

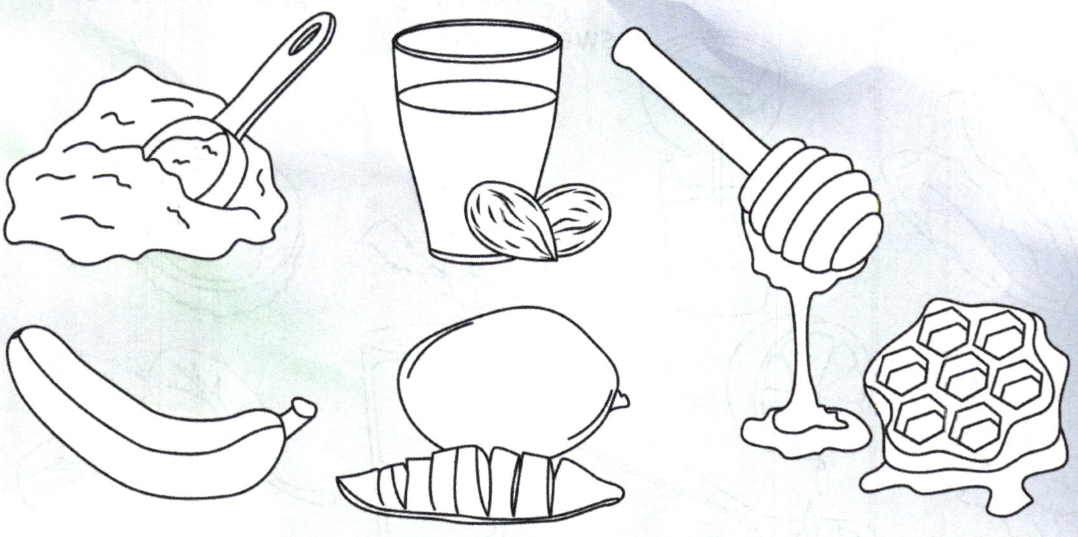

Liquid meals reduce irritation and help flush out processed food residues. Digestion becomes lighter. You start feeling cleaner inside — no more food "hangovers" or sluggish afternoons.

Blueberry Smoothie:

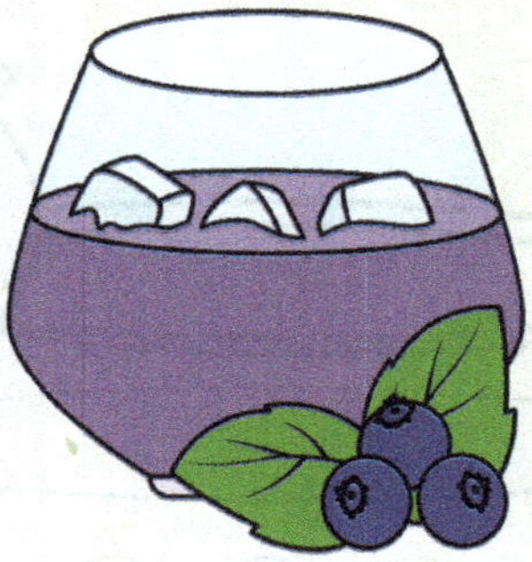

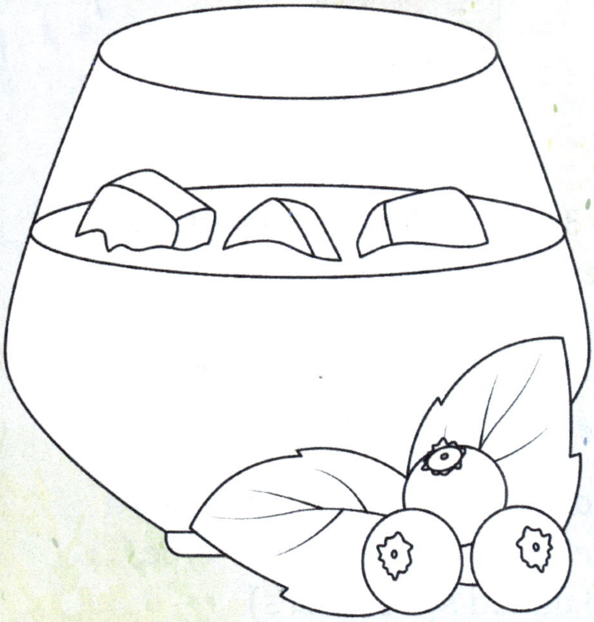

- 1 cup skim milk (or almond/milk of choice)
- $\frac{1}{2}$ cup vanilla-flavored yogurt (Greek or plant-based)
- 1 tsp vanilla powder (or $\frac{1}{2}$ tsp vanilla extract)
- 1 cup fresh or frozen blueberries

Optional: 1-2 tsp honey or maple syrup for extra sweetness

Calories~200-250 per serving (varies with milk, yogurt type, and added sweeteners).

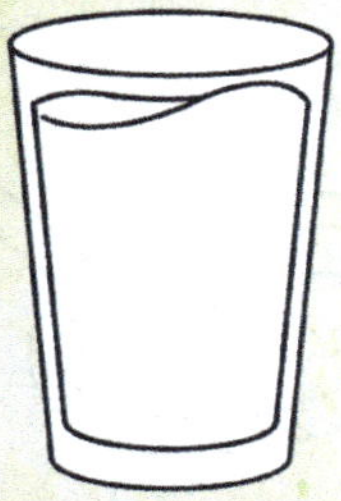

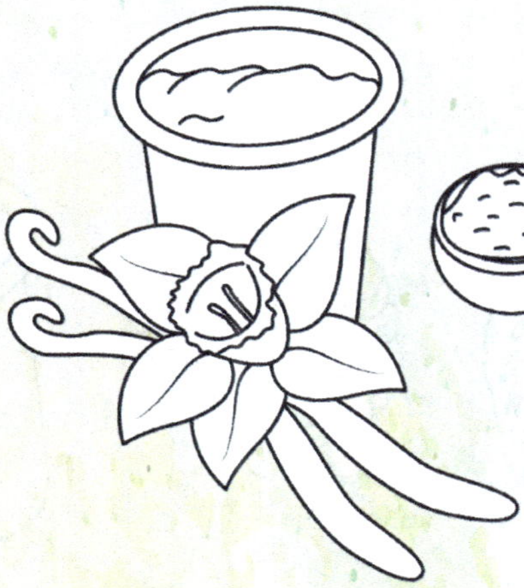

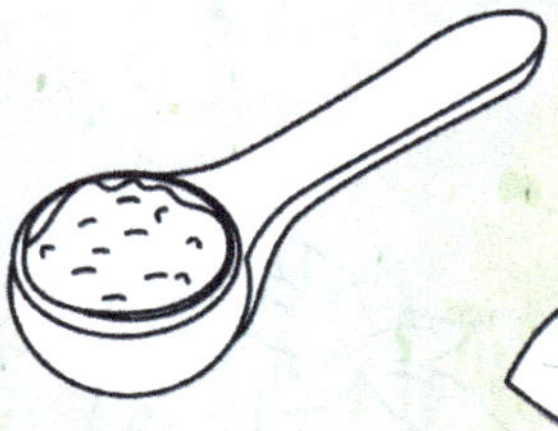

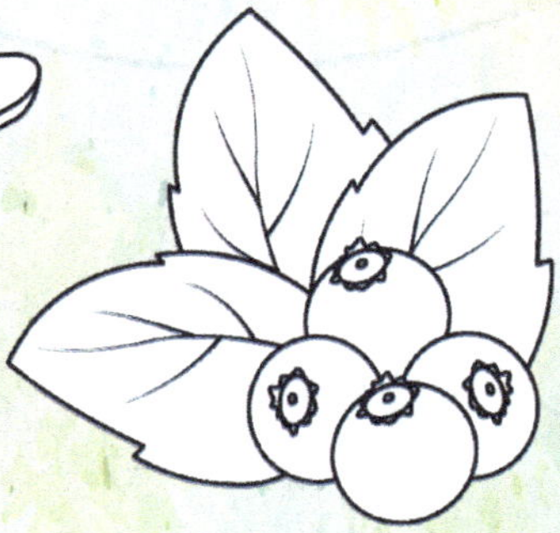

Day 3 - Gut Microbiome Support

Smoothies replace breakfast and lunch, protein-rich dinner.

Berry Detox Smoothie:

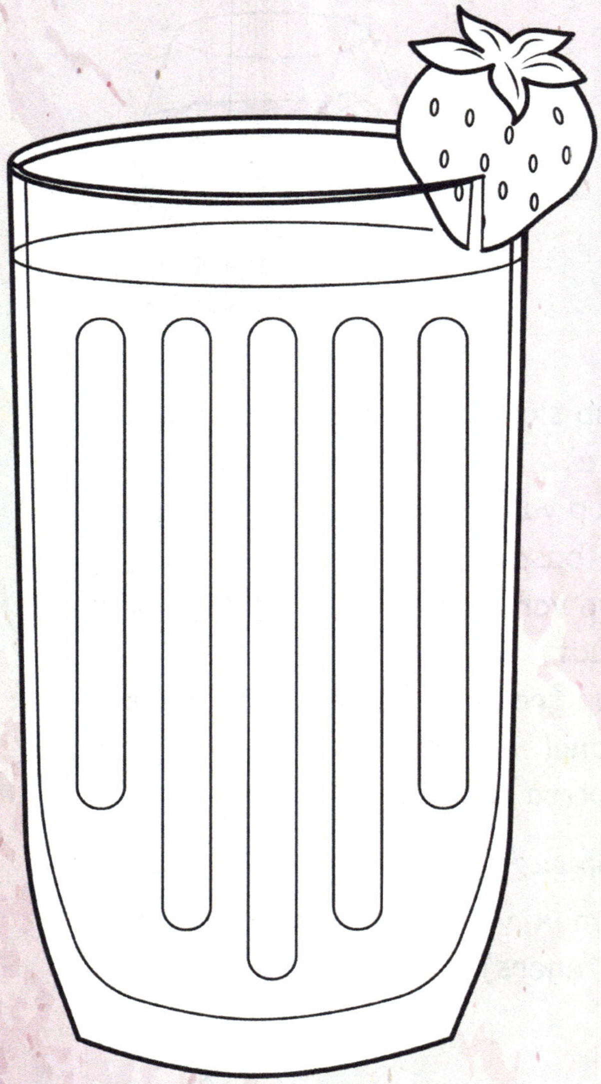

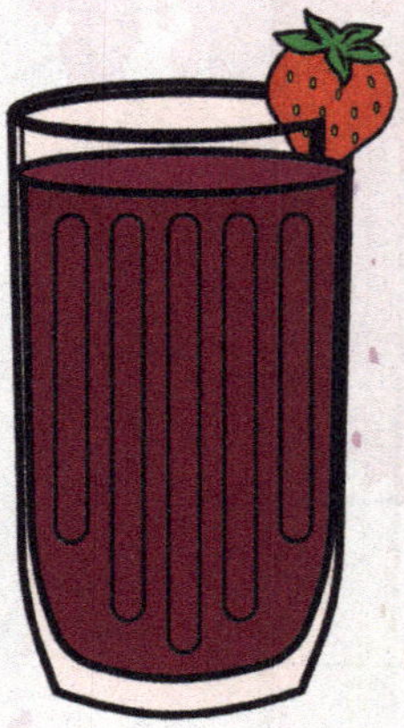

- 1/3 cup peeled + chopped raw beet (organic when possible)
- 1 cup frozen strawberries
- 1 cup frozen Raspberries
- 2/3 cup Greek yogurt

Calories~200-250 per serving (varies with milk, yogurt type, and added sweeteners).

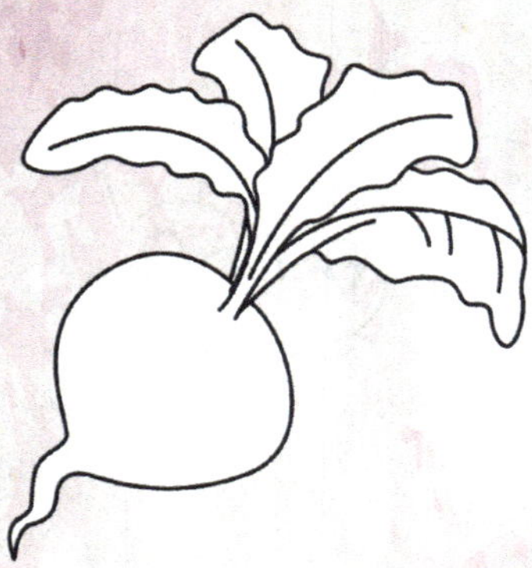

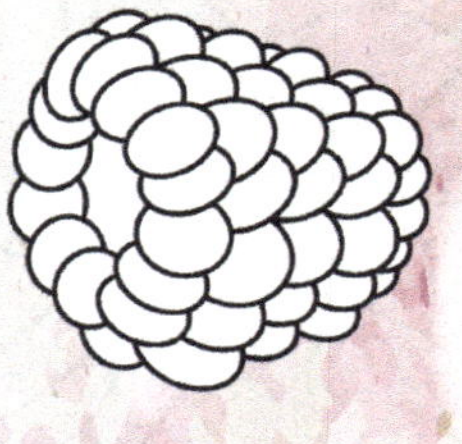

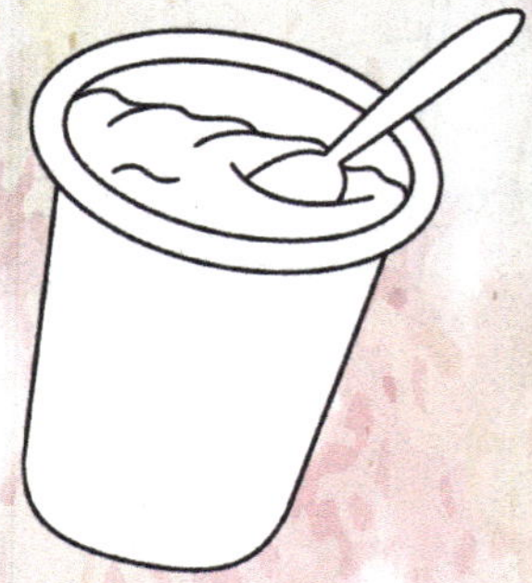

Your digestive system finds rhythm. The fiber and nutrients from smoothies begin to gently feed the good gut bacteria. Gas, irregularity, or discomfort noticeably decrease.

Creamy Banana Goodness:

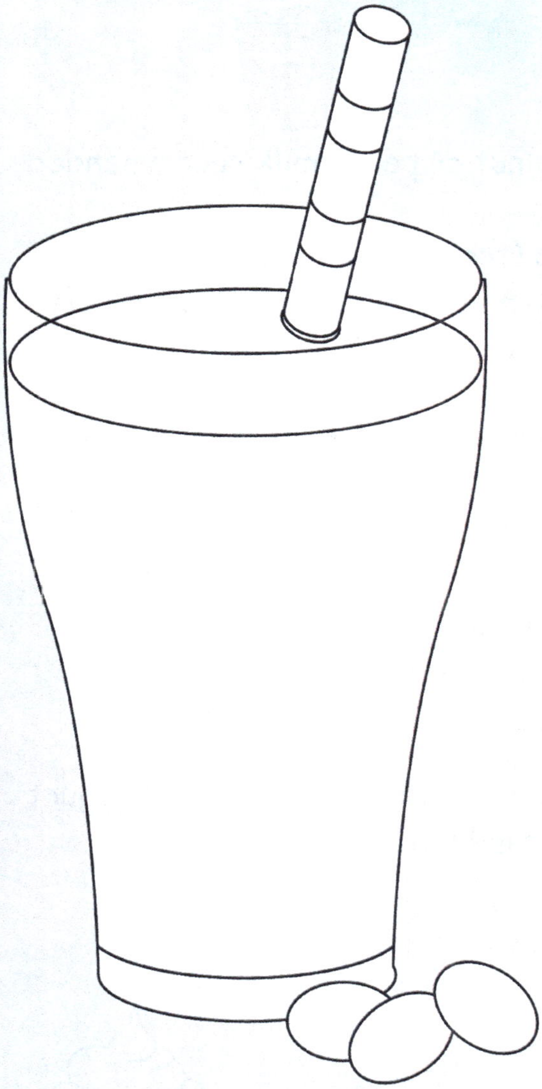

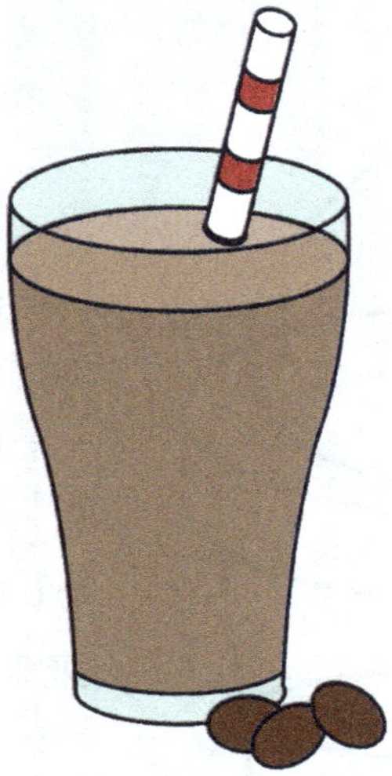

- 200 g banana (net weight without peel);
- 200 ml almond milk;
- 1 tsp cocoa;
- 1 tbsp almond butter;

Calories~200-250 per serving (varies with milk, yogurt type, and added sweeteners).

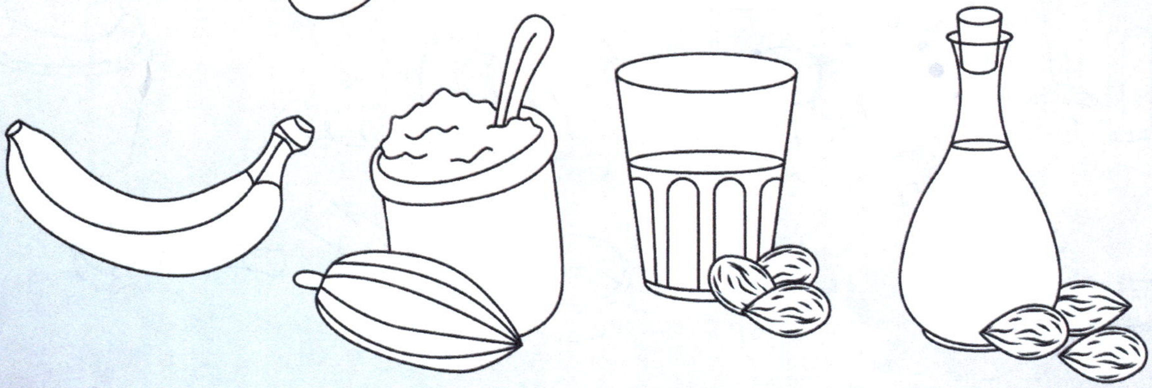

Day 4 - Clean Energy

Smoothies replace breakfast and lunch, protein-rich dinner.

Sweet Potato Carrot Pie Smoothie:

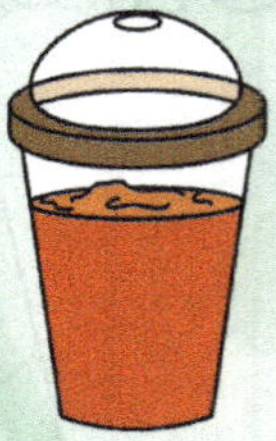

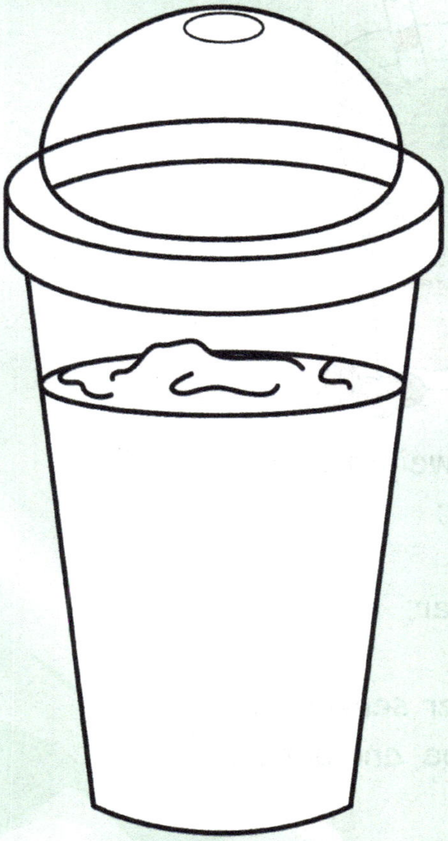

- $\frac{1}{2}$ cup nut milk (walnut or pecan milk recommended for richness)
- $\frac{1}{2}$ cup carrot juice (fresh or store-bought)
- $\frac{1}{2}$ cup roasted sweet potato (cooled; peel removed)
- 1 small whole carrot, chopped (or $\frac{1}{4}$ cup pre-shredded)
- $\frac{1}{4}$ cup Greek yogurt (or coconut milk yogurt for vegan)
- $\frac{1}{2}$ tsp vanilla extract
- $\frac{1}{4}$ tsp cinnamon

Pinch of nutmeg and ginger
1-2 tsp honey (optional, to taste)
Handful of ice cubes

Calories~250-350 per serving (depending on yogurt type, honey, and nut milk used).

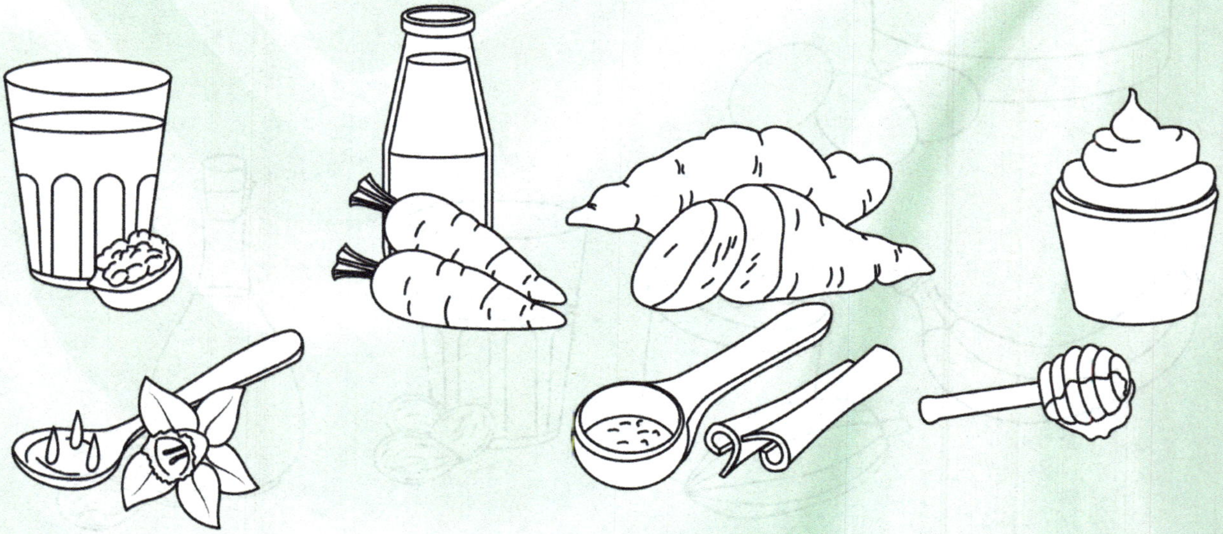

You feel energized and focused without the crash. No heavy digestion = no post-meal fatigue. Your stomach stays calm and light throughout the day. Evening protein supports deep sleep and muscle recovery.

Anti-Inflammatory Smoothie:

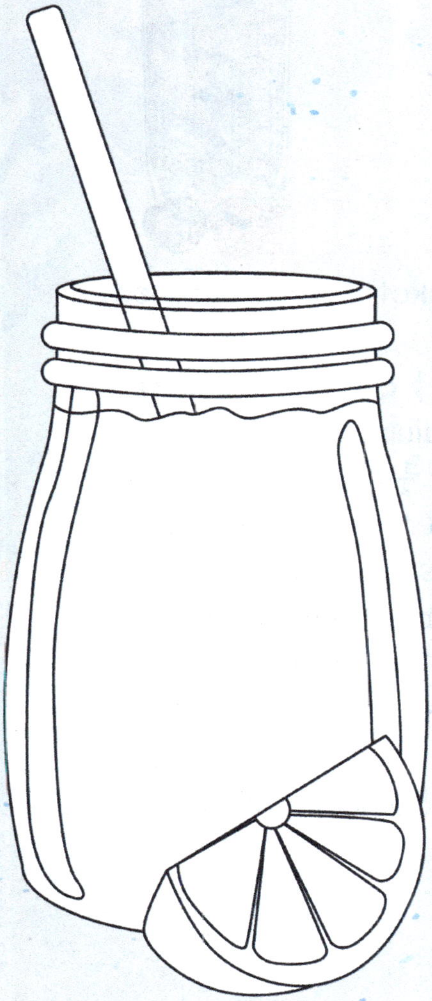

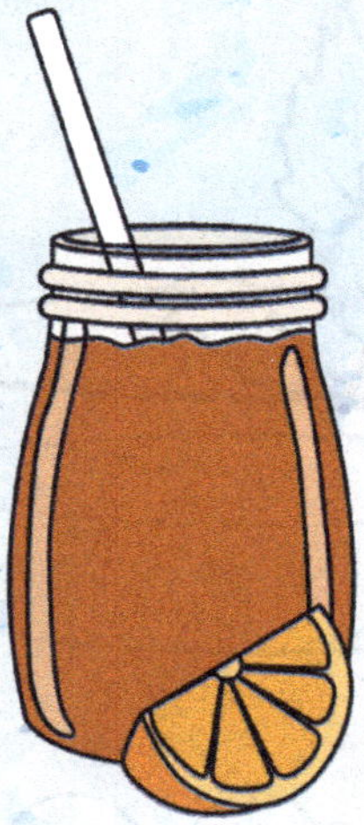

- 1 large ripe banana (previously peeled, sliced and frozen // more for a sweeter smoothie)
- 1 cup fresh orange juice
- 1/2 Tbsp fresh ginger (peeled // 1 small knob yields ~1/2 Tbsp)
- 1/2 cup carrot juice

Calories~200-250 per serving (varies with milk, yogurt type, and added sweeteners).

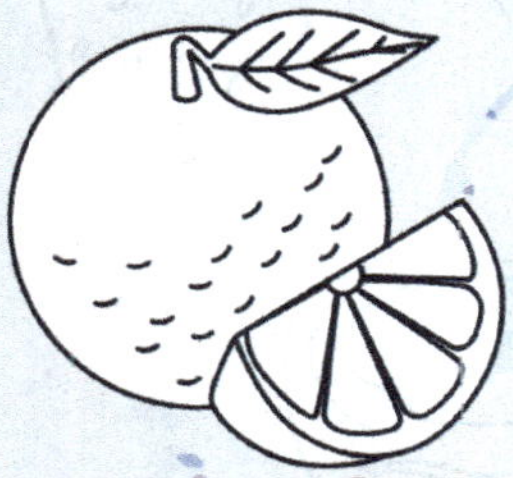

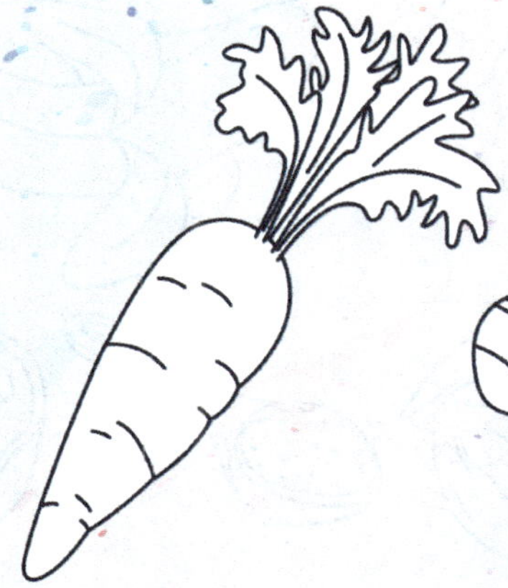

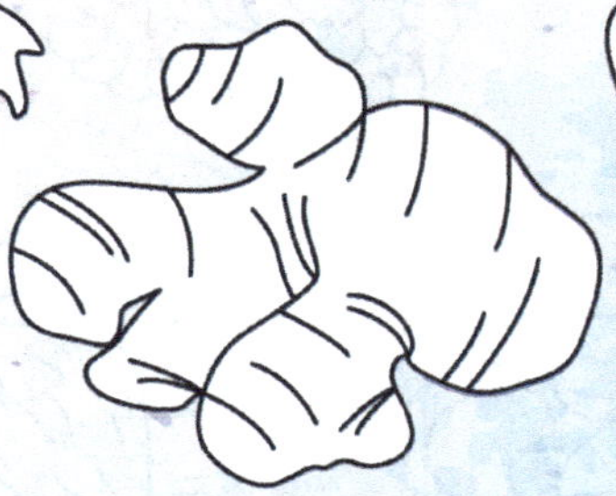

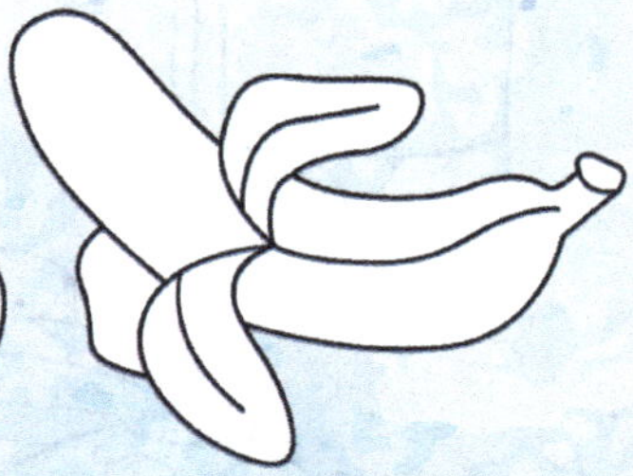

Day 5 – Inflammation Calms Down

Smoothies replace breakfast and lunch, protein-rich dinner.

Brain Power:

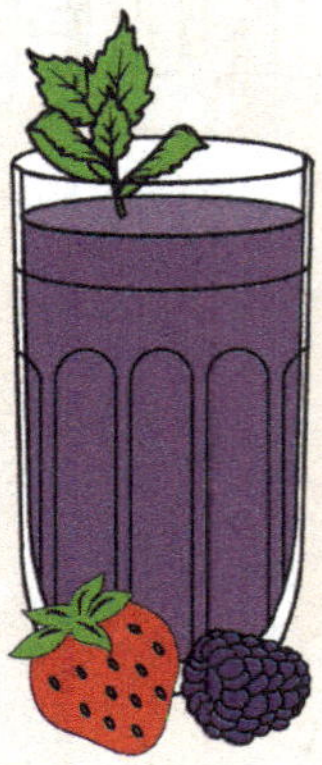

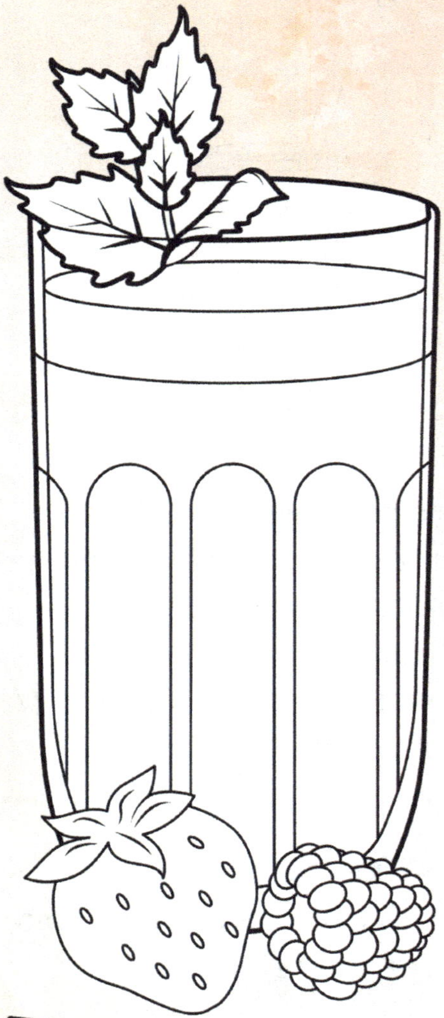

- Acai puree packet: 1 (unsweetened) (anthocyanins)
- Blackberries: $\frac{1}{2}$ cup (manganese)
- Banana: $\frac{1}{2}$ medium (energy base)
- Strawberries: $\frac{1}{2}$ cup (fisetin)
- Goji berries: 1 tbsp (zeaxanthin)
- Almonds: 1 tbsp (vitamin E)
- Chia seeds: 1 tbsp (omega-3s)
- Coconut milk: 1 cup (MCTs)
- Ice: $\frac{1}{2}$ cup

Calories~400-450 per serving.

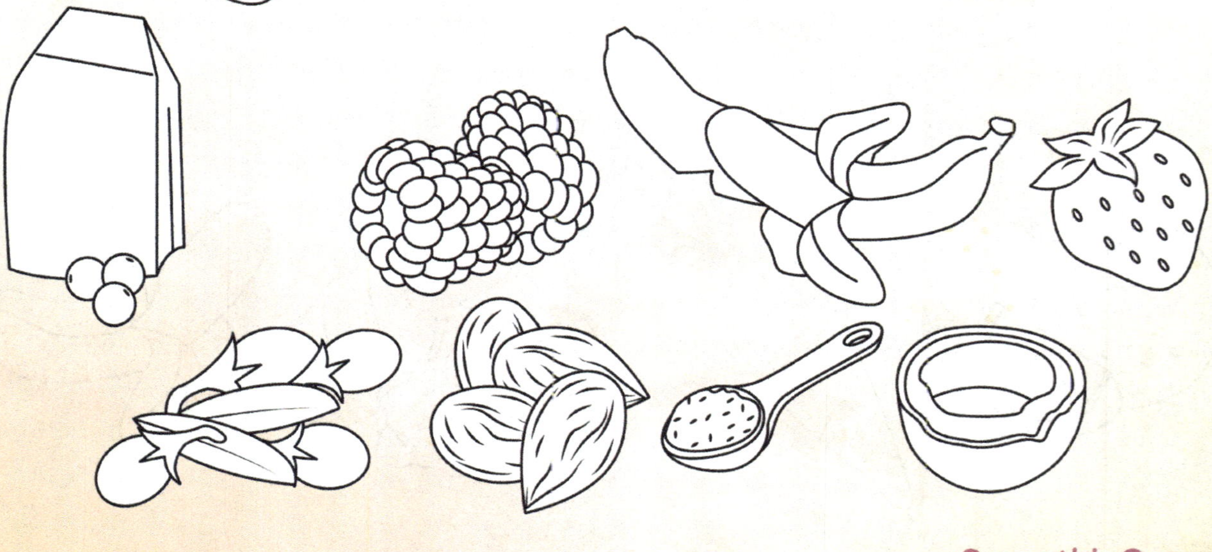

With irritants like processed fats and sugars gone, the digestive lining begins to heal. If you've experienced gastritis, acid reflux, or bloating before — symptoms ease. The body absorbs nutrients more efficiently.

Antioxidant Boosting Power:

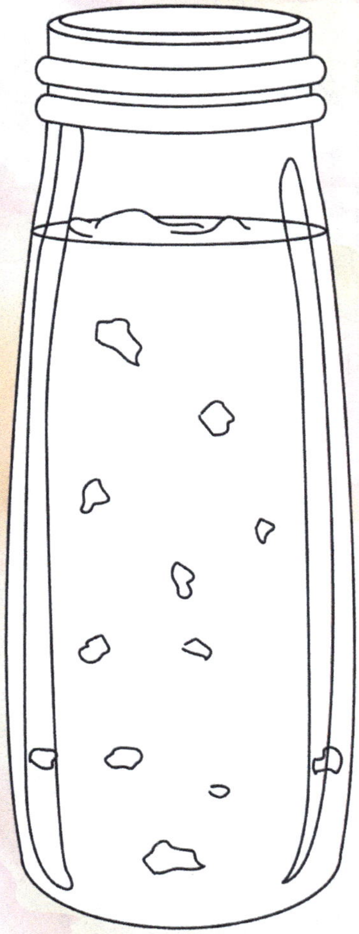

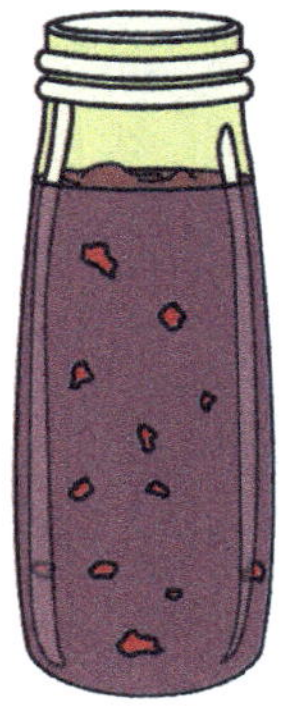

- Wild blueberries: 1 cup
- Strawberries: $\frac{1}{2}$ cup
- Banana: $\frac{1}{2}$ medium (potassium base)
- Greek yogurt: 1 scoop ($\frac{1}{4}$ cup) (probiotics)
- Chia seeds: 1 tbsp (soaked) (omega-3s)
- Pomegranate juice: $\frac{1}{2}$ cup
- Brewed green tea: $\frac{1}{2}$ cup (catechins)
- Ice: $\frac{1}{2}$ cup

Calories~300-320 per serving (varies with milk, yogurt type, and added sweeteners).

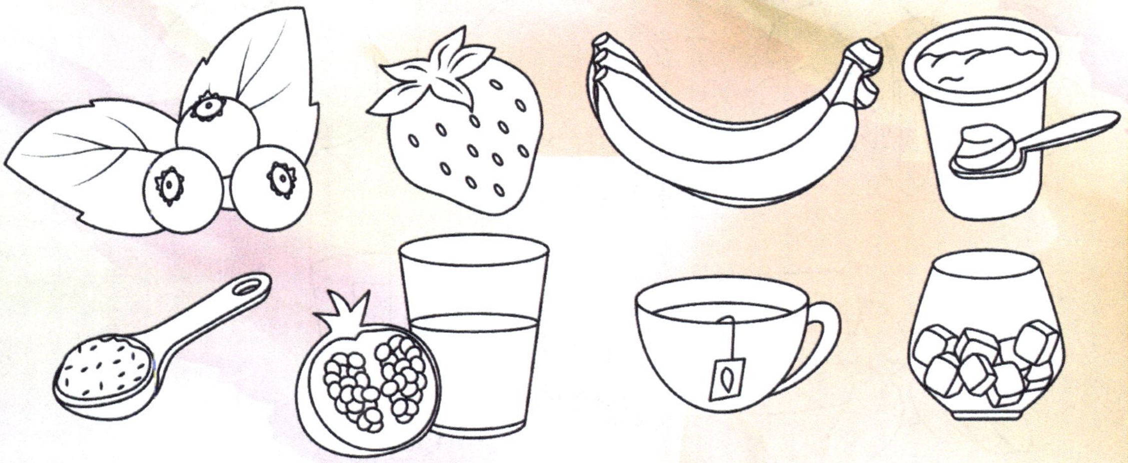

Day 6 – Noticeable Lightness
Smoothies replace breakfast and lunch, protein-rich dinner.

Spinach and Mango Smoothie:

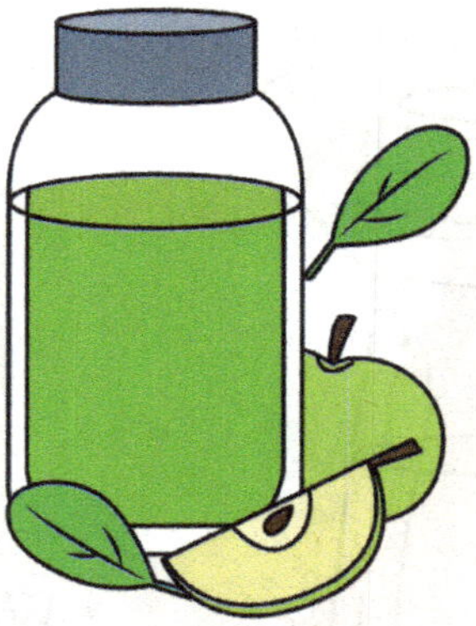

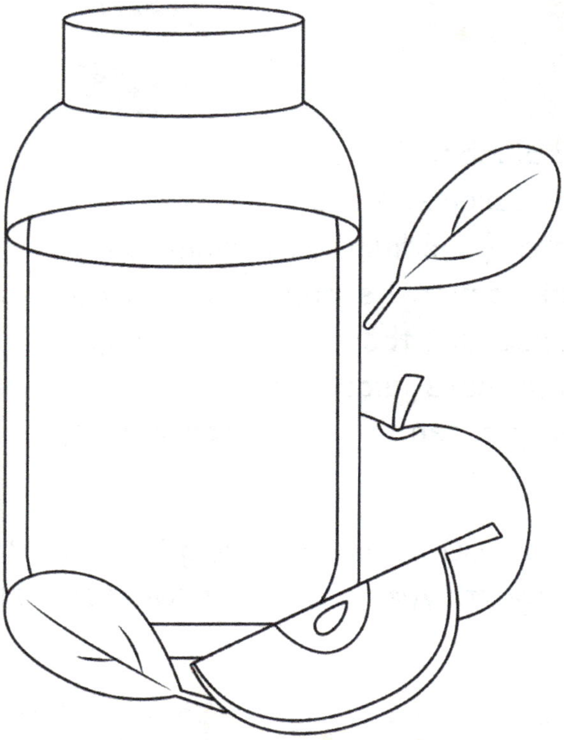

- 1 cup spinach
- $\frac{1}{2}$ mango
- $\frac{1}{2}$ green apple
- $\frac{1}{2}$ banana
- $\frac{1}{2}$ cup plant-based milk

Calories: ~160

Benefits: High in fiber, vitamins A/C, and natural sweetness for digestion.

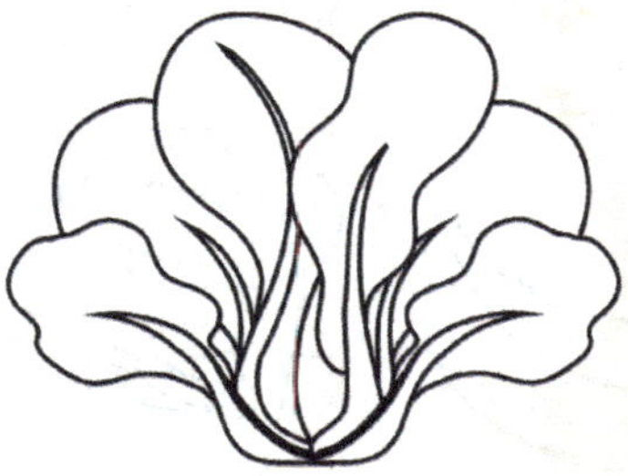

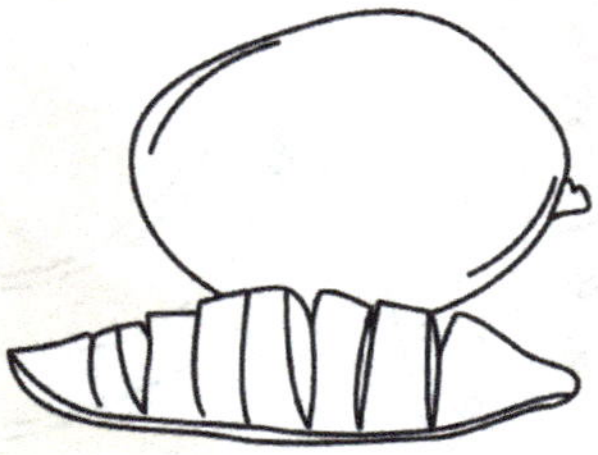

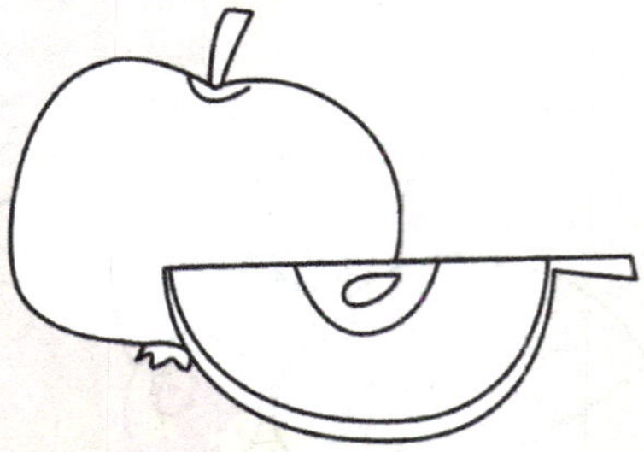

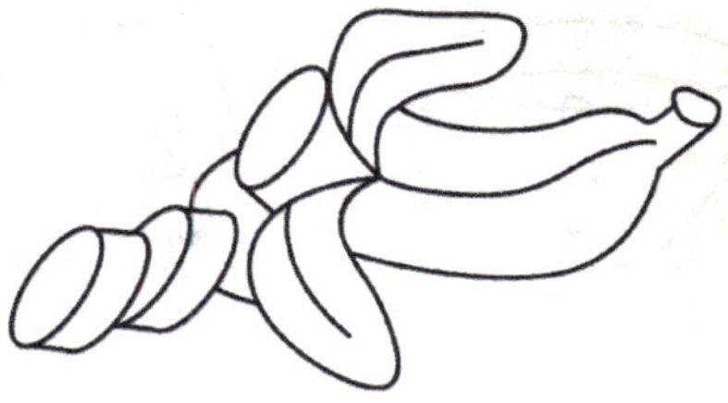

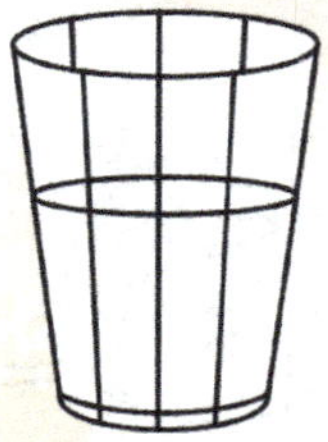

The stomach and gut work smoothly and predictably. You feel physically lighter, mentally clearer, and emotionally more stable. No more heaviness, cramping, or unpredictable hunger spikes.

Green Fat Burner:

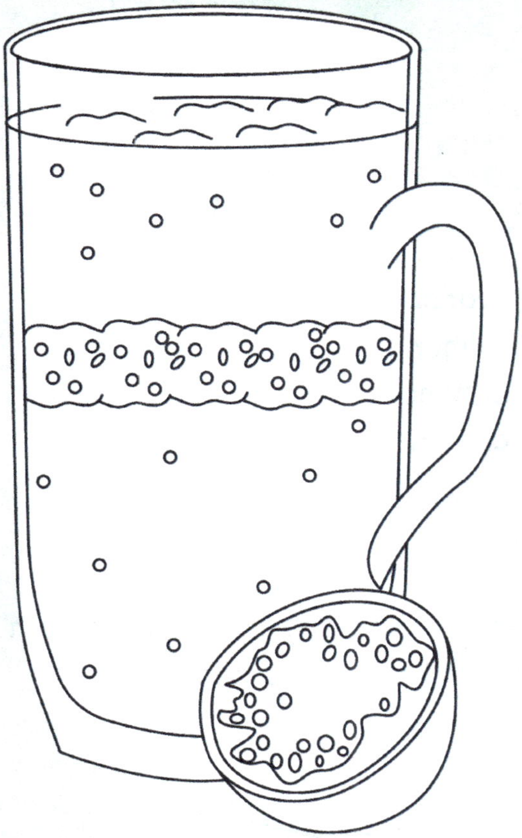

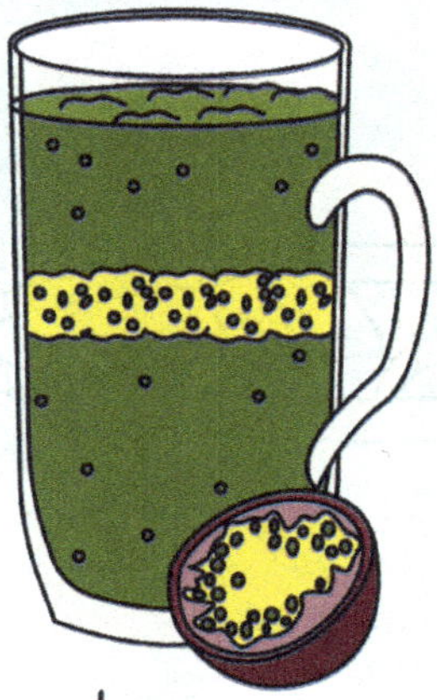

- $\frac{1}{2}$ cucumber
- 2 passion fruits (pulp)
- 1 cup kale/spinach
- $\frac{1}{2}$ green apple
- $\frac{1}{4}$ cup apple juice

Calories: ~150

Benefits: Hydrating, rich in vitamin C and electrolytes.

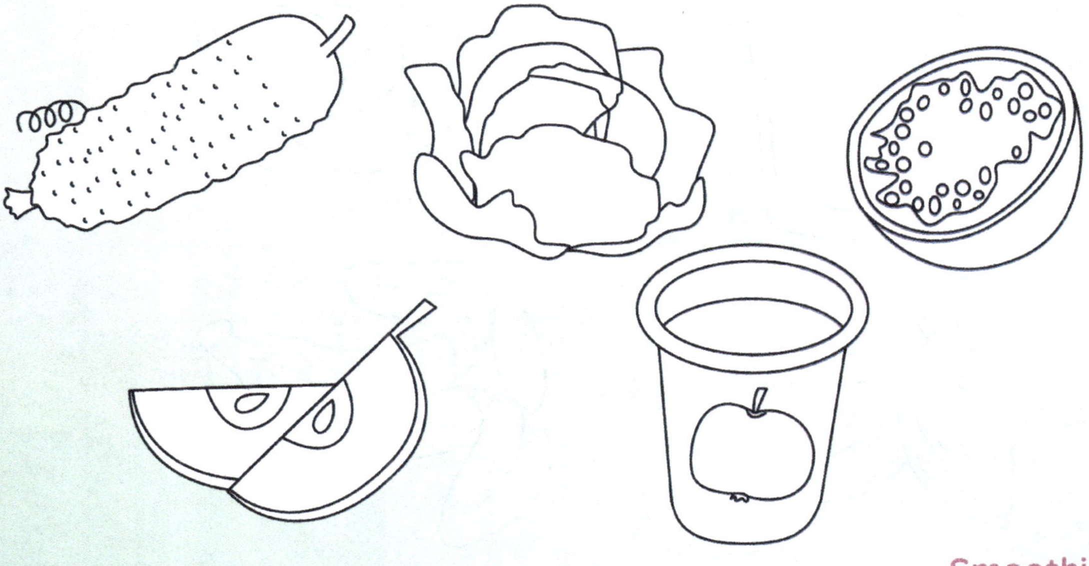

Day 7 – Digestive Balance

Smoothies replace breakfast and lunch, protein-rich dinner.

Avocado and Almond Smoothie:

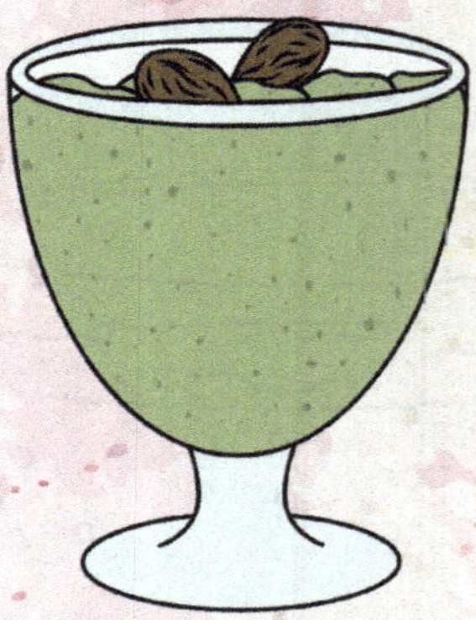

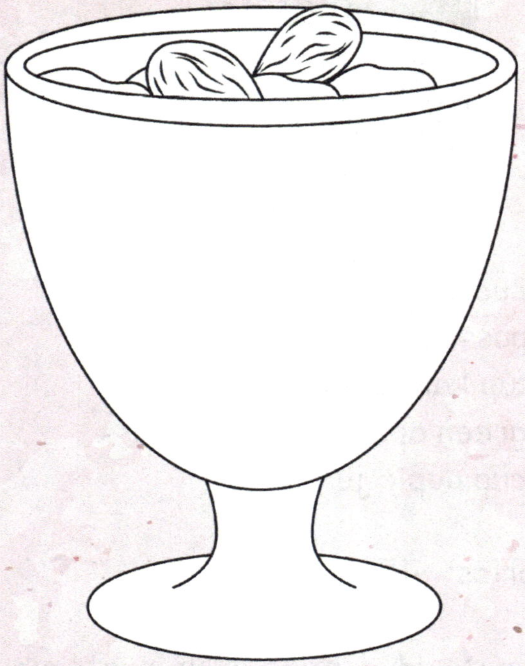

- $\frac{1}{4}$ avocado
- 10 almonds
- $\frac{1}{2}$ banana
- $\frac{1}{2}$ cup nut milk

Calories: ~190

Benefits: Healthy fats and protein for skin health and energy.

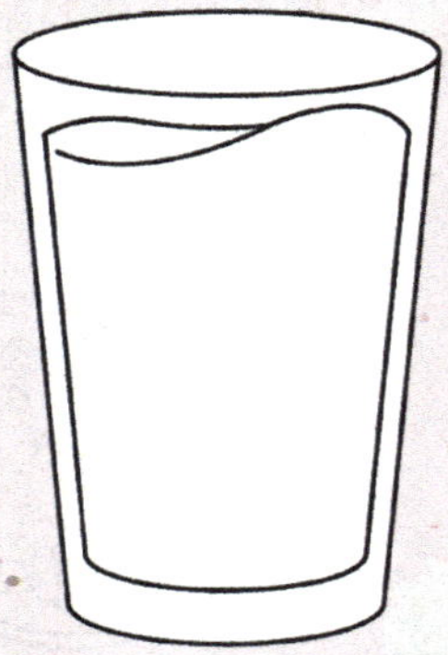

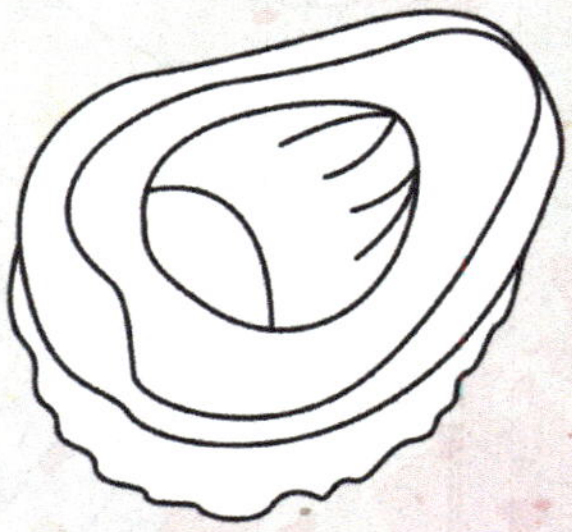

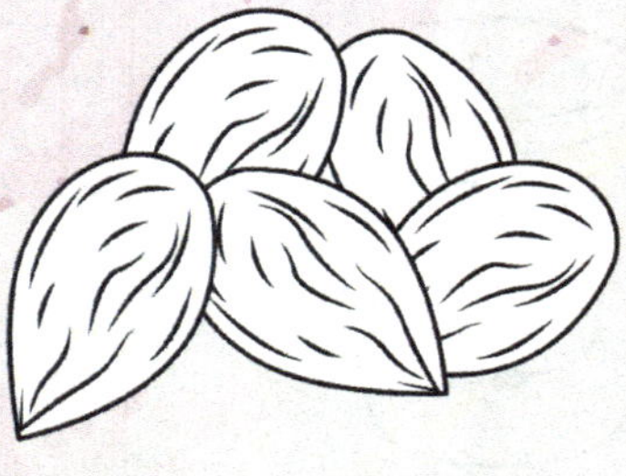

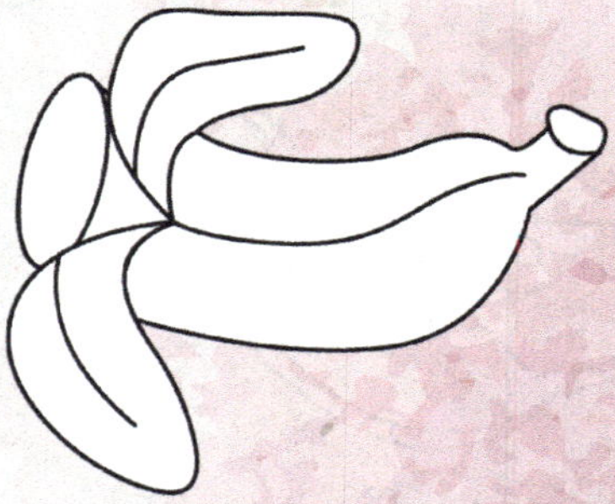

By now, your system has adapted. Your stomach handles food calmly and efficiently. The routine of light nourishment during the day and protein in the evening creates a sustainable digestive balance — with energy, comfort, and control.

Probiotic Digestion Boost:

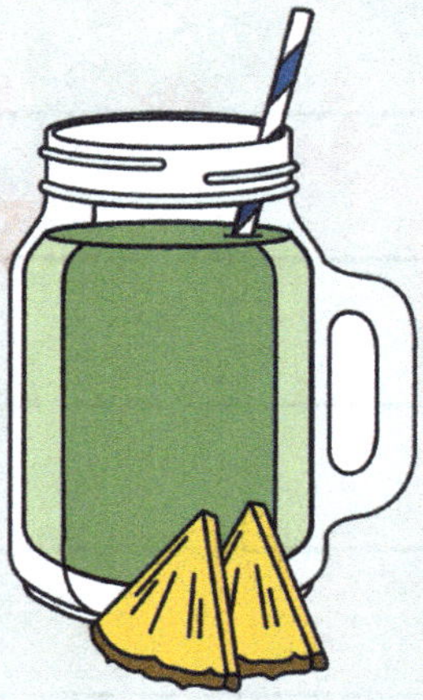

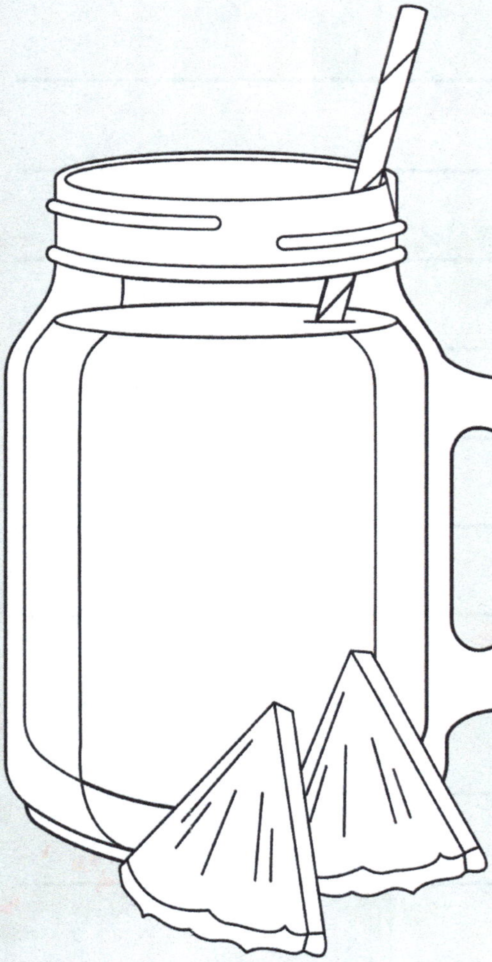

- $\frac{1}{2}$ cup pineapple
- $\frac{1}{2}$ green apple
- 1 cup spinach
- $\frac{1}{4}$ cup unsweetened yogurt
- $\frac{1}{4}$ cup nut milk/water

Calories: ~125

Benefits: Boosts immunity and digestion with probiotics.

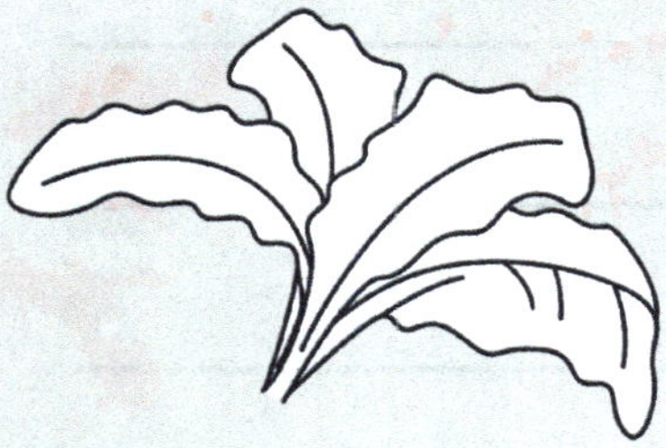
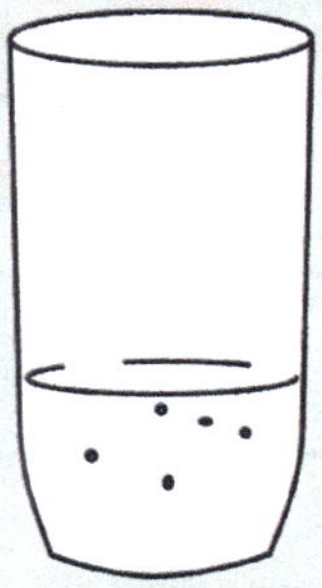
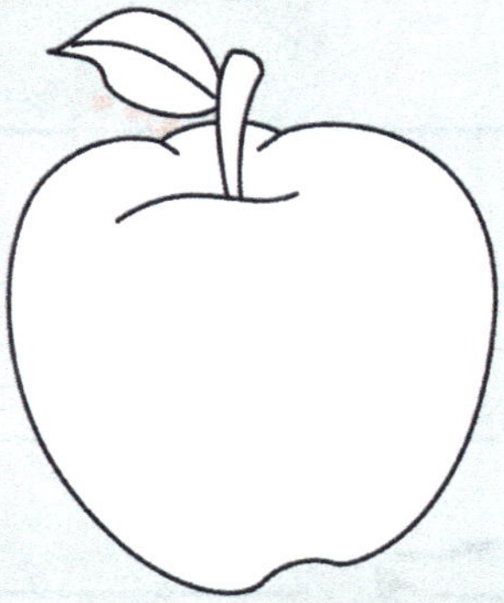
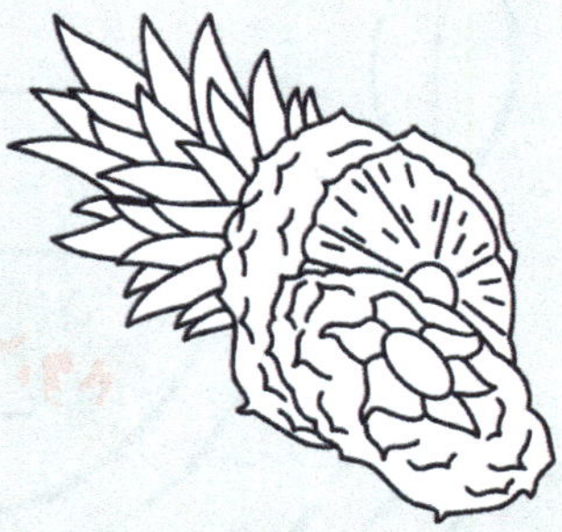

My Notes & Ideas

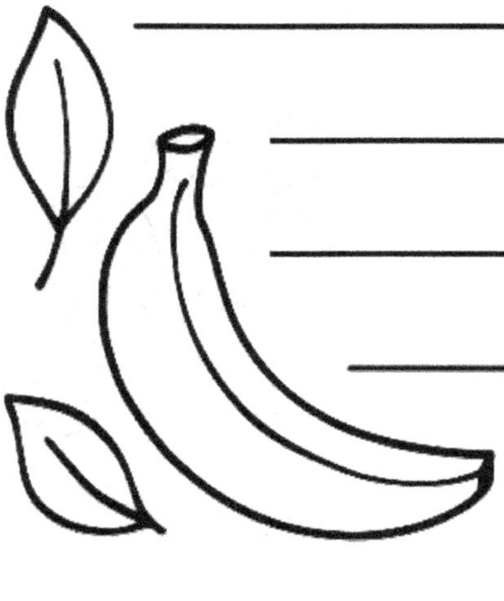

Weekly Wellness Check-In

Weight This Week ______________________

____

____

Favorite Smoothie ________________

____

____

Mood This Week ______________________

____

____

Notes ________________________

____

Day 8 - New Rhythm

Smoothie at 10:00 AM and 6:00 PM.

Banana and Peanut Butter Smoothie:

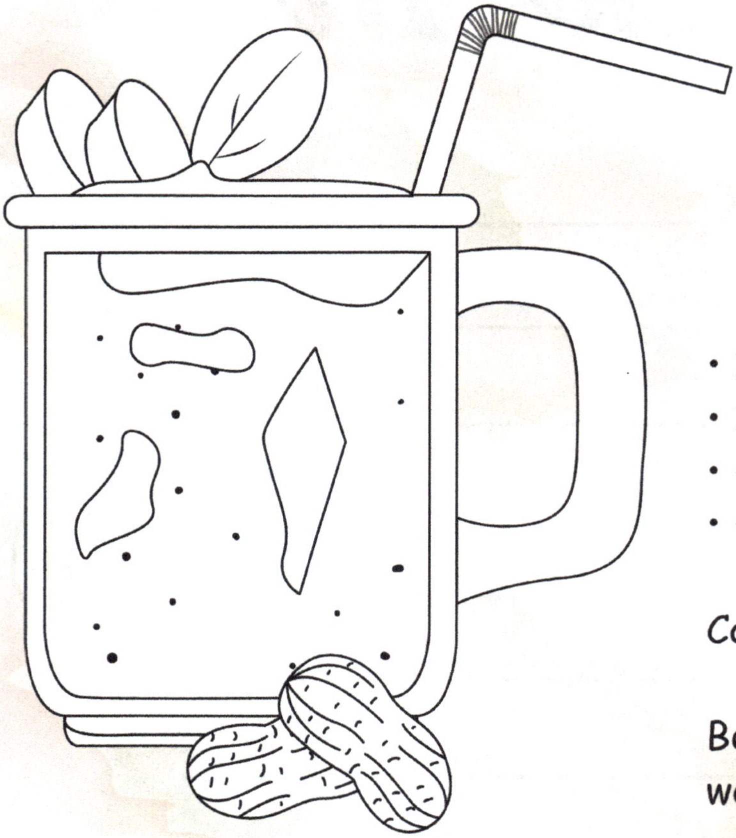

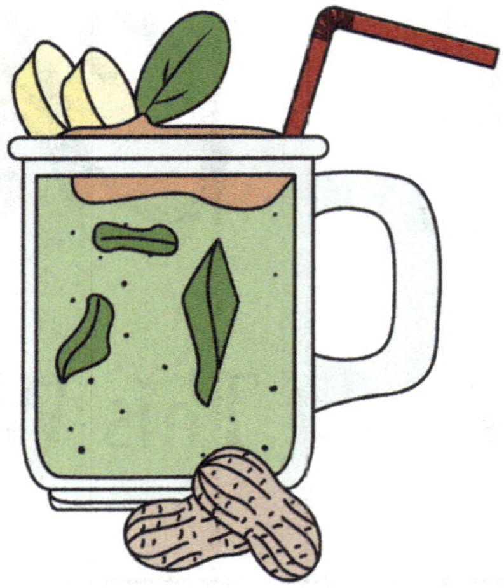

- 1 banana
- 1 tbsp peanut butter
- ½ cup spinach
- ½ cup low-fat milk

Calories: ~250

Benefits: Energy-dense for workouts and muscle recovery.

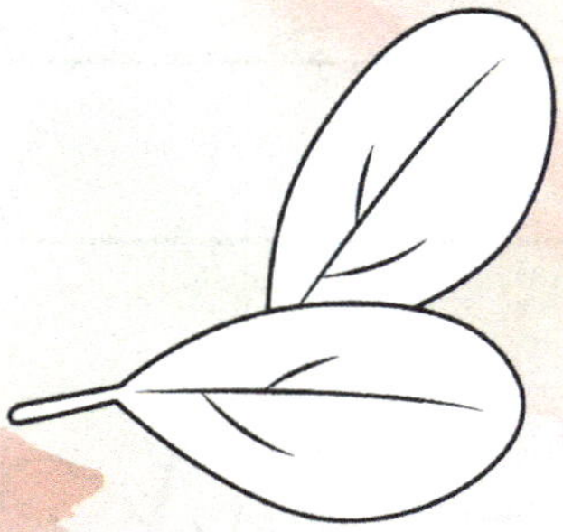

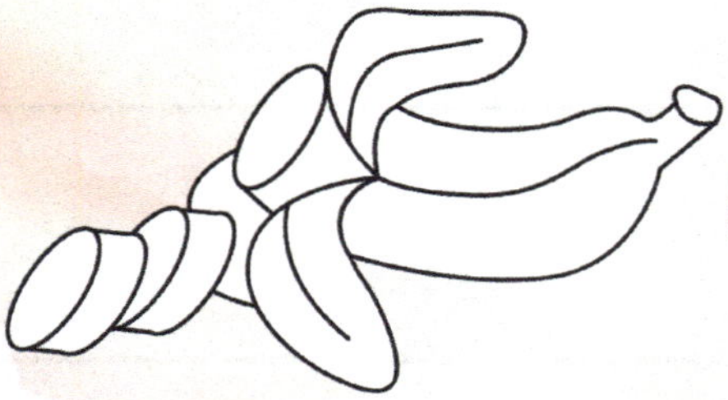

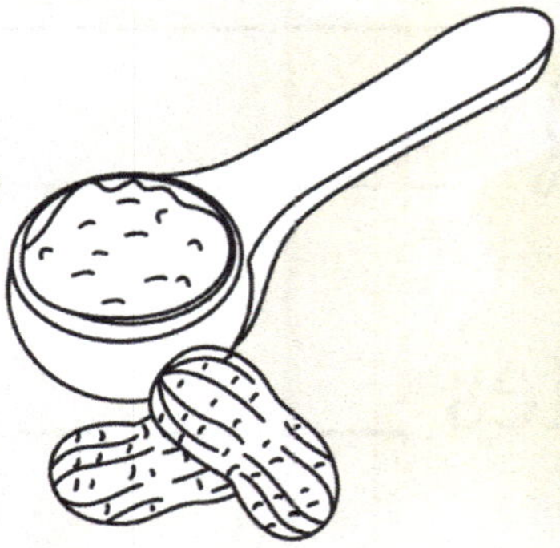

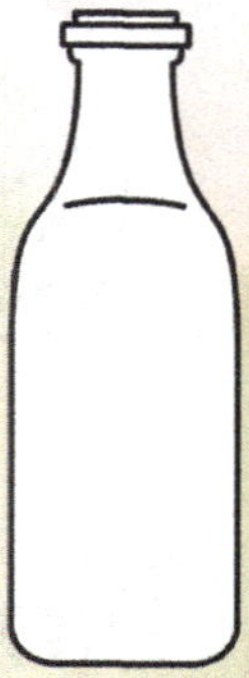

Your body adjusts to a more spaced-out eating pattern. Hunger signals stabilize. You feel light in the morning and grounded in the evening — without needing solid meals.

Immunity Booster Green Delight:

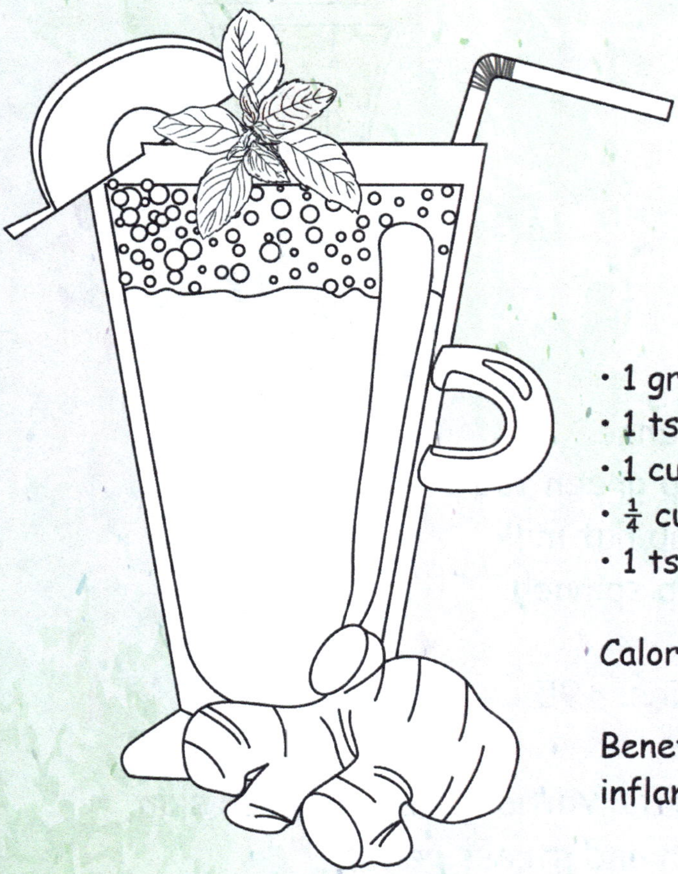

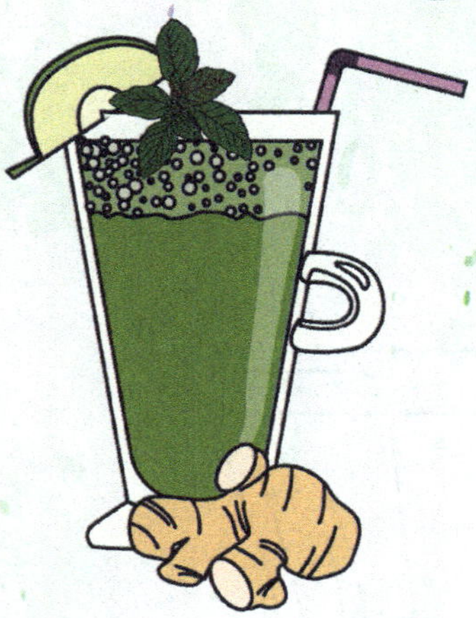

- 1 green apple
- 1 tsp fresh ginger
- 1 cup spinach
- $\frac{1}{4}$ cup unsweetened yogurt
- 1 tsp honey

Calories: ~150

Benefits: Detoxifies, reduces inflammation, and boosts immunity.

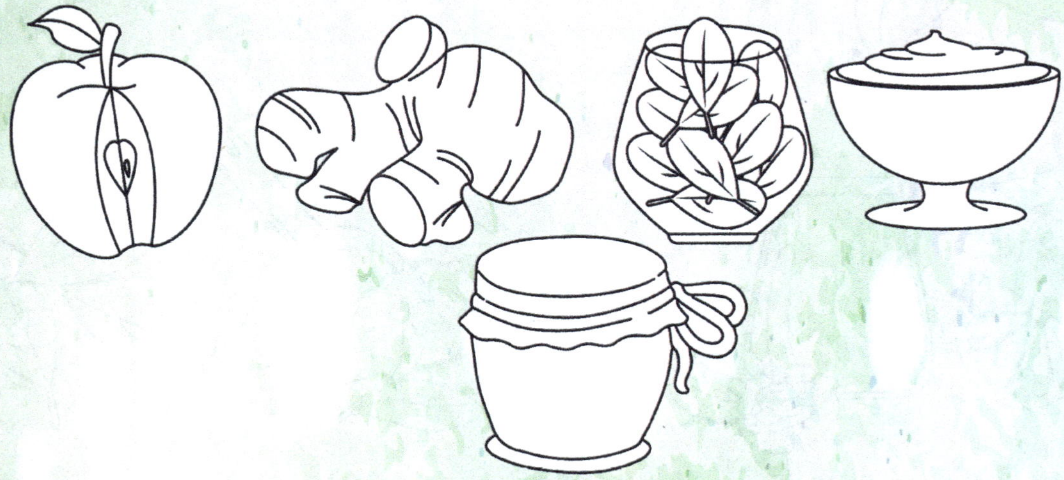

Day 9 - Deepened Detox
Smoothie at 10:00 AM and 6:00 PM.

Sunrise Pink Smoothie:

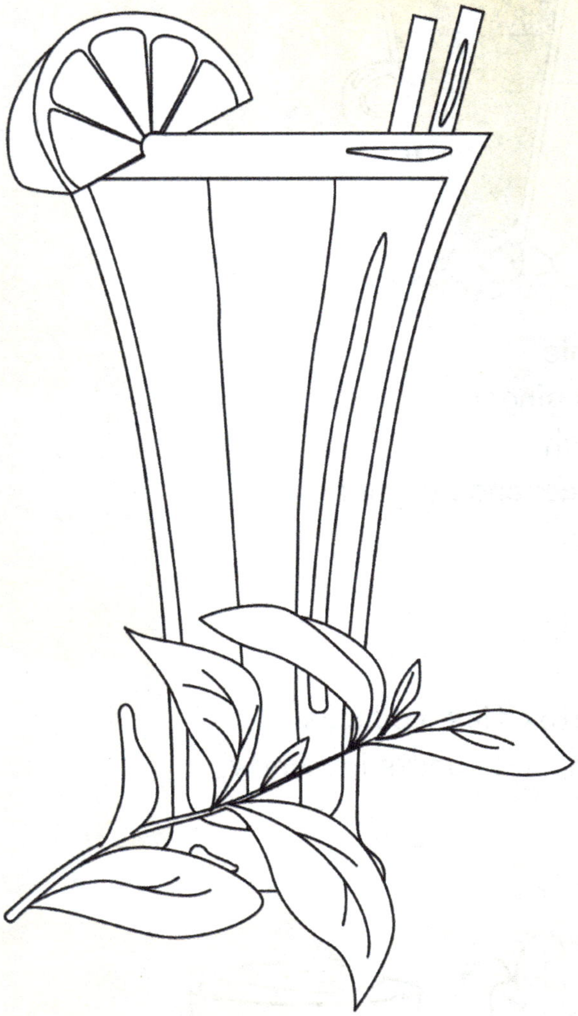

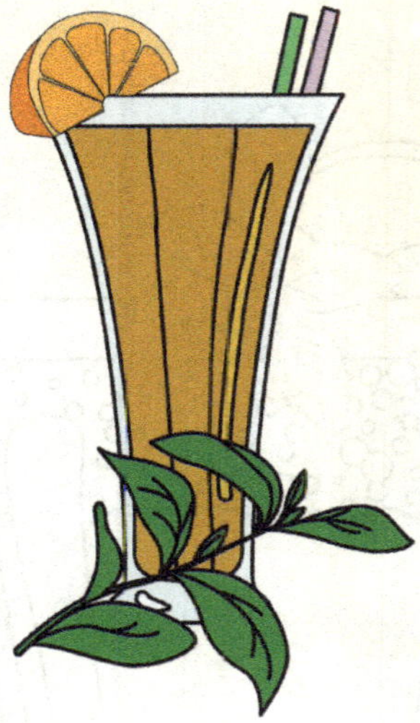

- 1 orange
- 1 tsp green tea powder
- ½ cup nut milk
- 1 cup spinach

Calories: ~95

Benefits: Antioxidant-rich for skin health and stress relief.

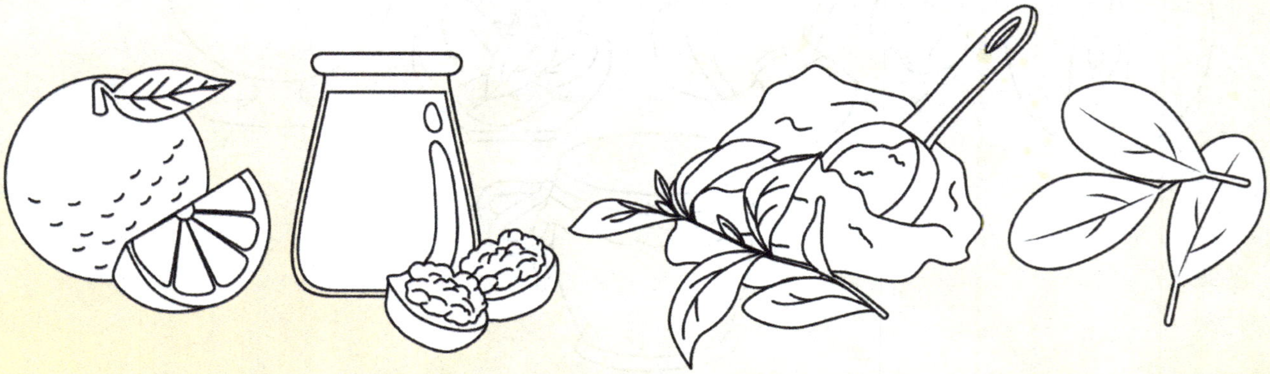

The longer gaps between meals give your digestive system even more rest. Cleansing processes deepen, especially in the liver and gut. Skin and eyes may look clearer.

Strawberry and Chia Seed Smoothie:

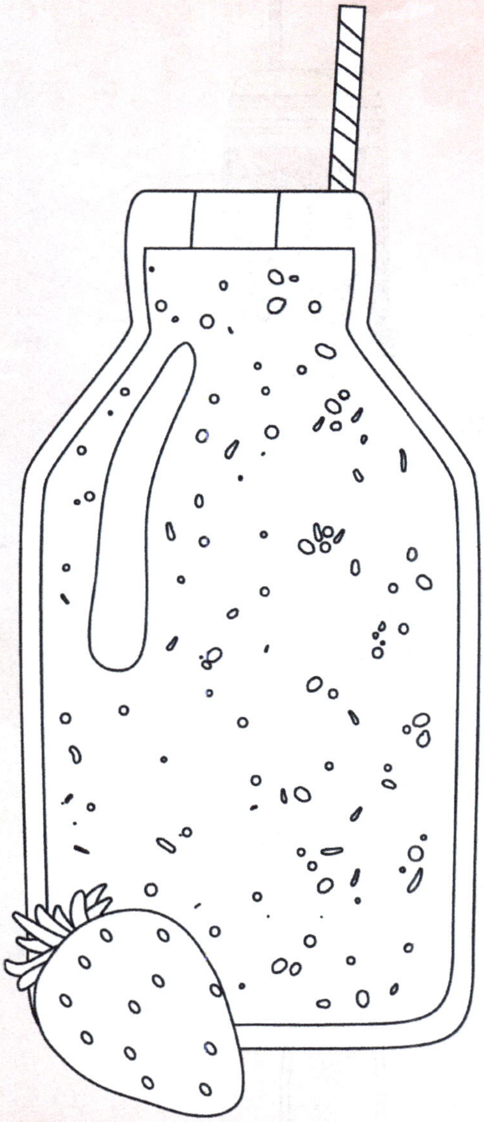

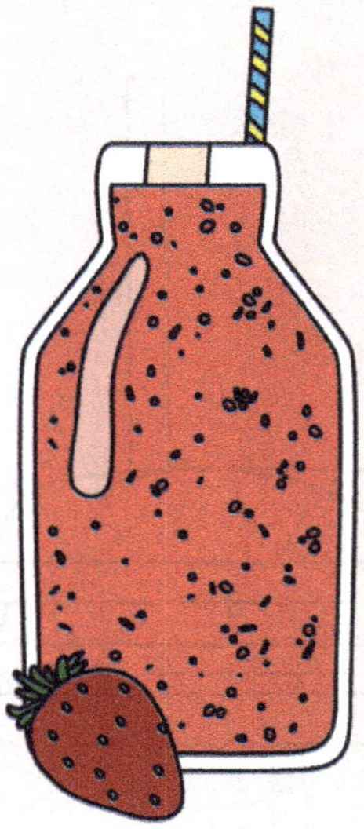

- 1 cup strawberries
- 1 tsp chia seeds
- $\frac{1}{2}$ cup almond milk
- 1 tsp honey

Calories: ~110

Benefits: Supports skin and digestion with Omega-3s and vitamin C.

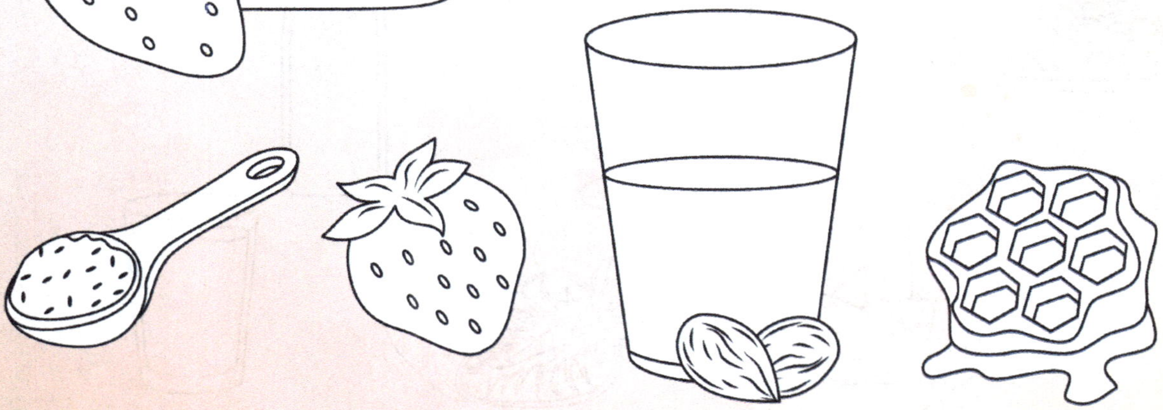

Day 10 – Stronger Gut Resilience

Smoothie at 10:00 AM and 6:00 PM.

Immunity Boost Smoothie:

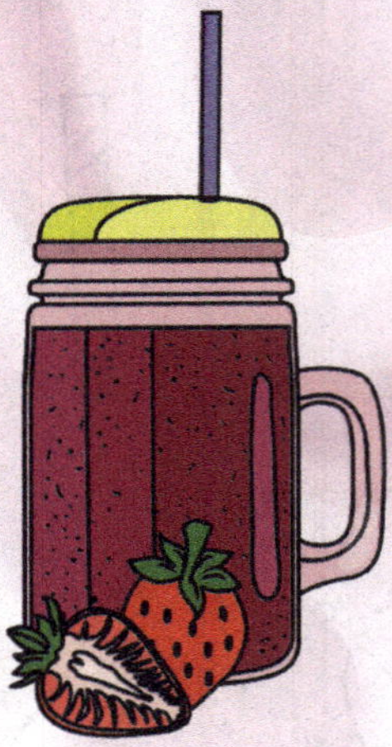

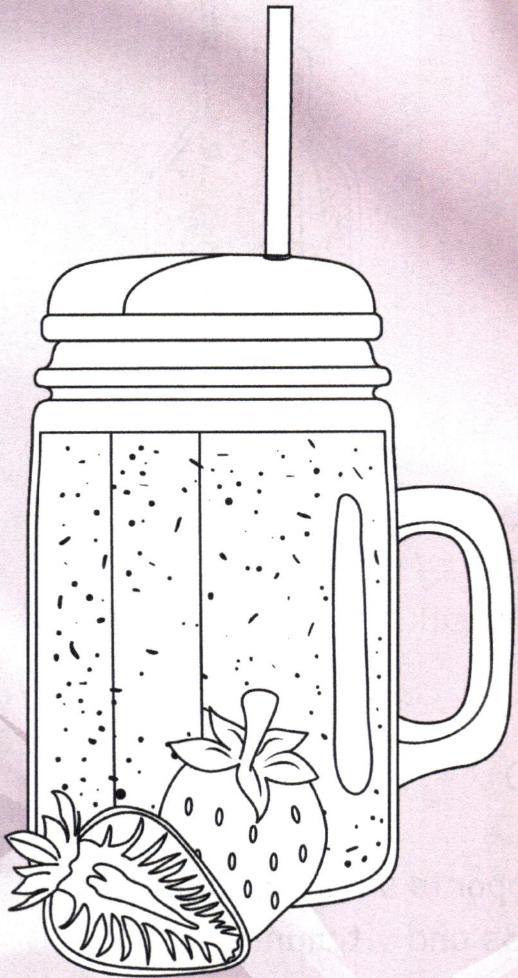

- 1 frozen banana
- $\frac{1}{4}$ cup old-fashioned oats
- $\frac{1}{2}$ cup frozen spinach
- $\frac{1}{2}$ cup filtered water
- $\frac{1}{2}$ cup frozen strawberries
- $\frac{1}{2}$ cup plain unsweetened kefir

Calories: ~350

Benefits: Boosts immune system with probiotics and high fiber content.

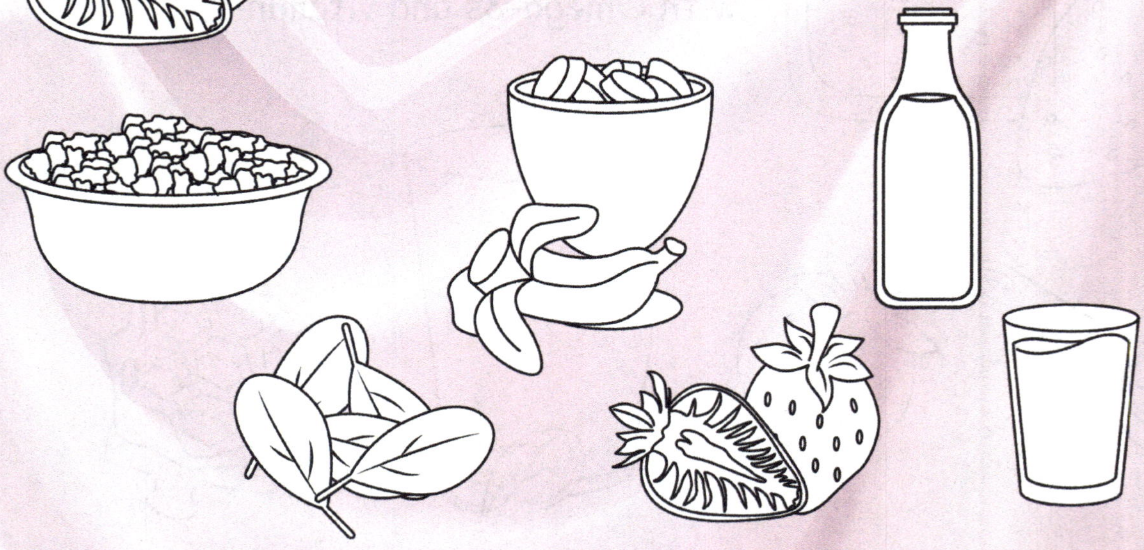

Your gut lining strengthens, and your microbiome continues to thrive. No bloating, no urgency. Your digestion feels quiet, controlled, and efficient.

Sweet Satisfaction Smoothie:

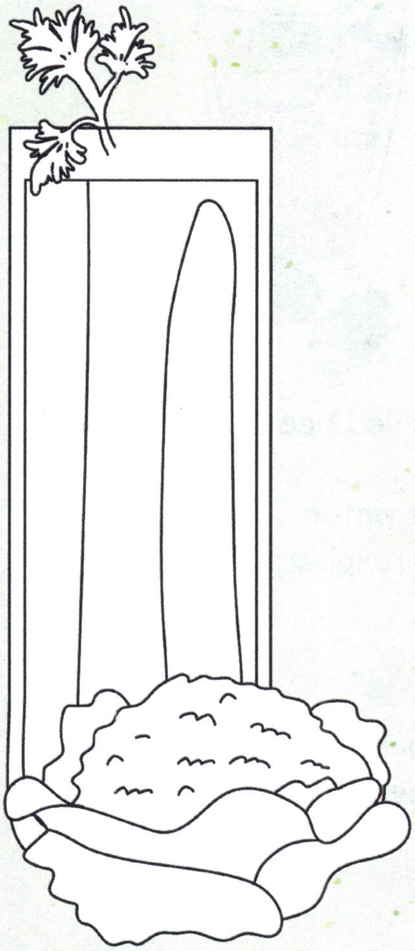

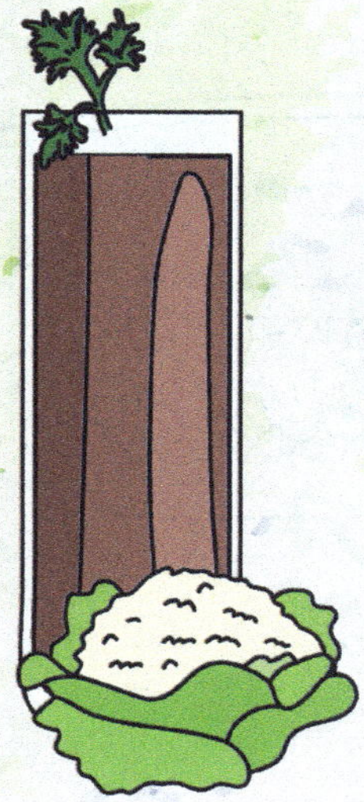

- ½ cup frozen riced cauliflower
- 2 tbsp peanut powder
- 1 frozen banana
- 1 cup 2% milk
- 1 tbsp dark cocoa powder

Calories: ~270

Benefits: Fulfills sweet cravings without compromising clean eating.

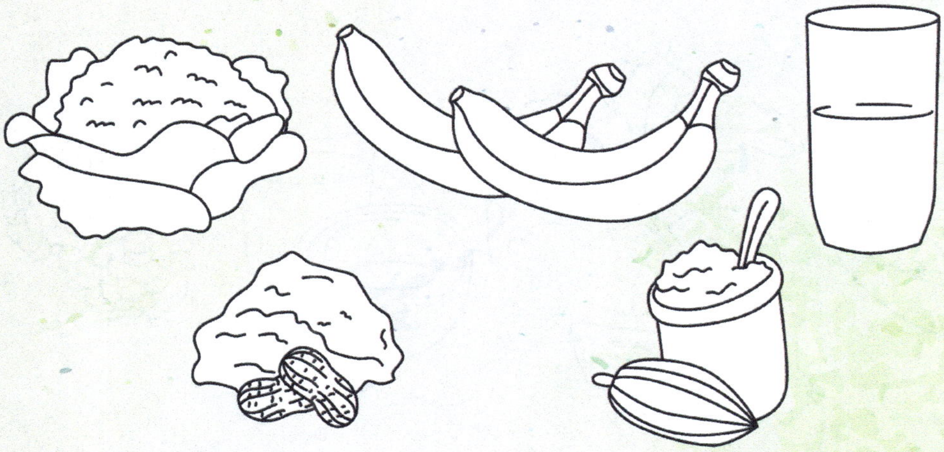

Day 11 – Metabolic Reset

Smoothie at 10:00 AM and 6:00 PM.

Turn Up the Beet Smoothie:

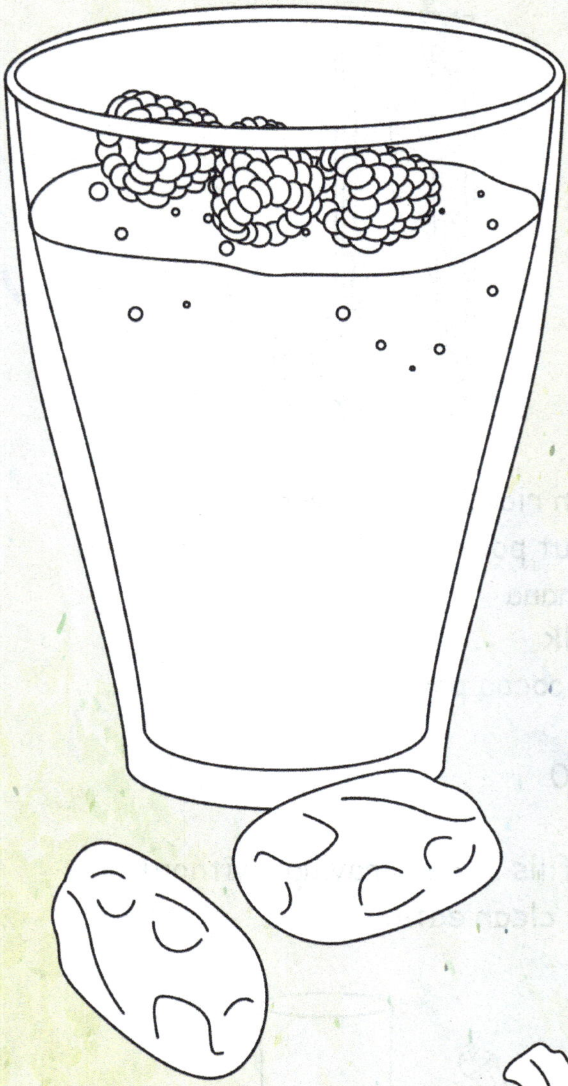

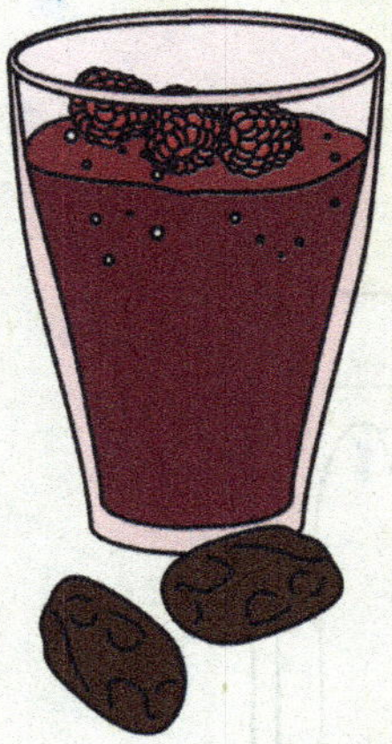

- $\frac{1}{2}$ cup cooked red beet (1 small beet)
- 1 pitted date
- 1 cup coconut water
- $\frac{1}{2}$ cup frozen raspberries

Calories: ~210

Benefits: Supports energy with beets and raspberries, enhances hydration.

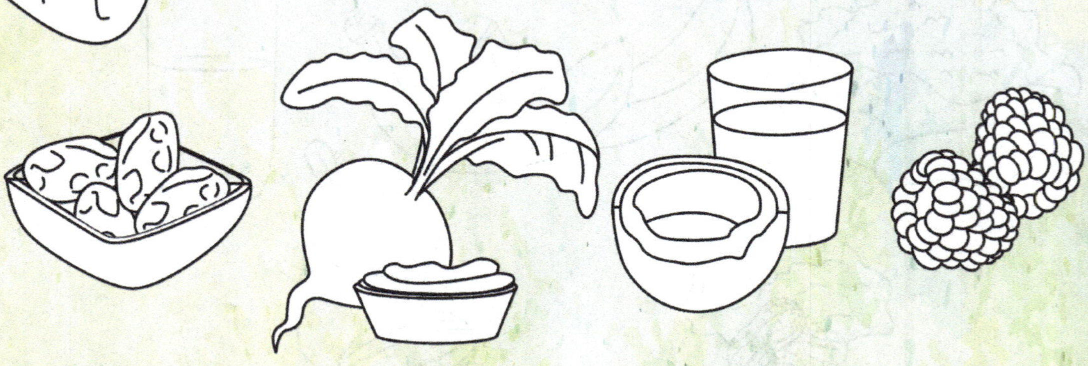

With fewer insulin spikes and consistent nutrients, your metabolism starts to rebalance. You feel more in sync with your natural hunger. Energy stays smooth throughout the day.

Avocado Burner Smoothie:

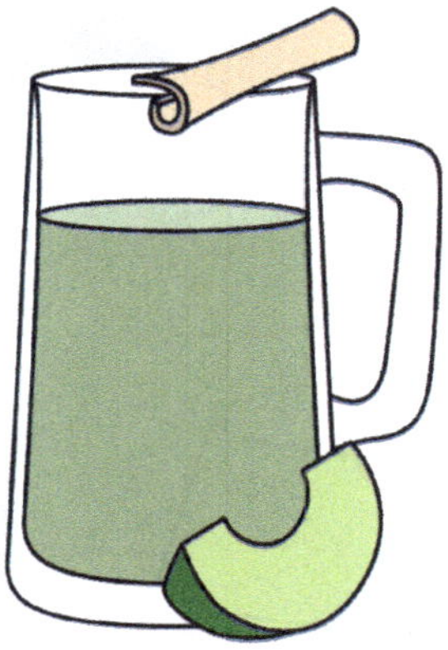

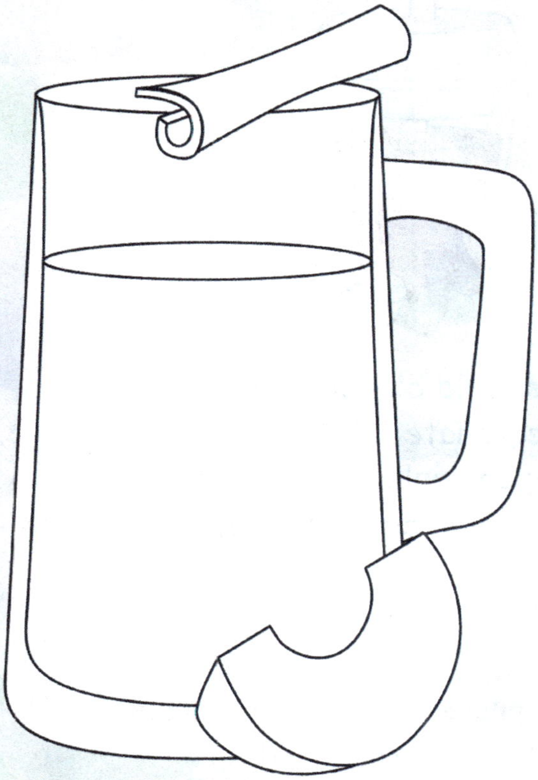

- $\frac{1}{2}$ medium avocado
- 1 pitted date
- 1 frozen banana
- $\frac{1}{2}$ tsp ground cinnamon
- $\frac{1}{2}$ cup filtered water
- $\frac{1}{2}$ cup unsweetened almond milk

Calories: ~320

Benefits: Promotes metabolism with avocado and cinnamon.

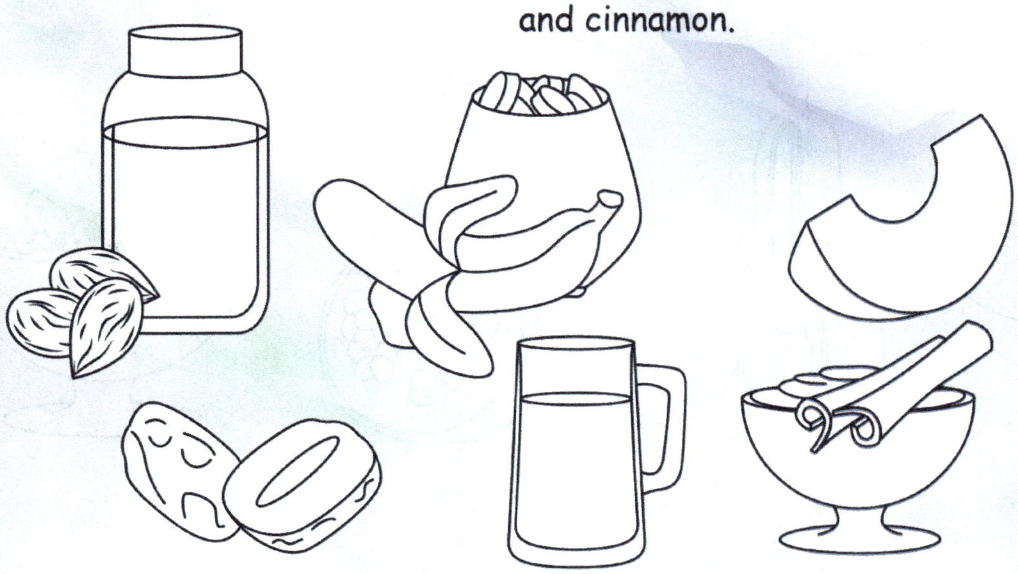

Day 12 - Mental Lightness
Smoothie at 10:00 AM and 6:00 PM.

Sunrise Pink Smoothie:

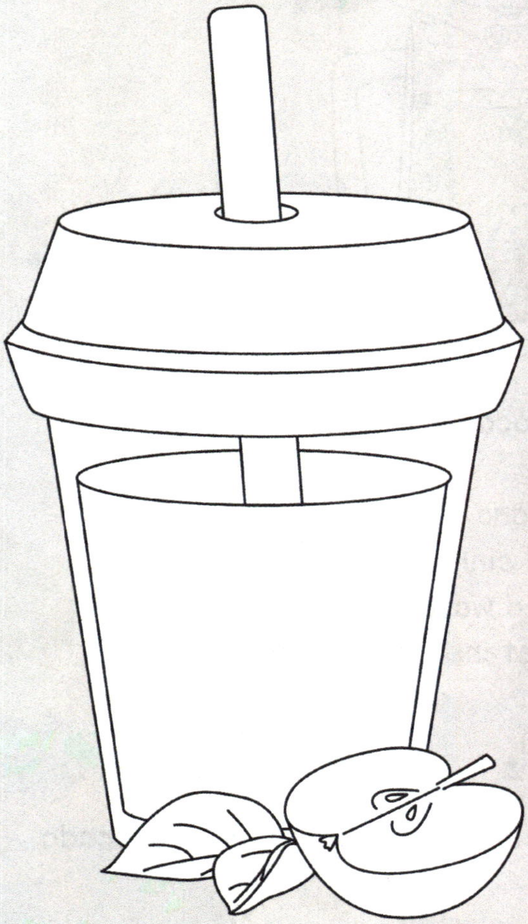

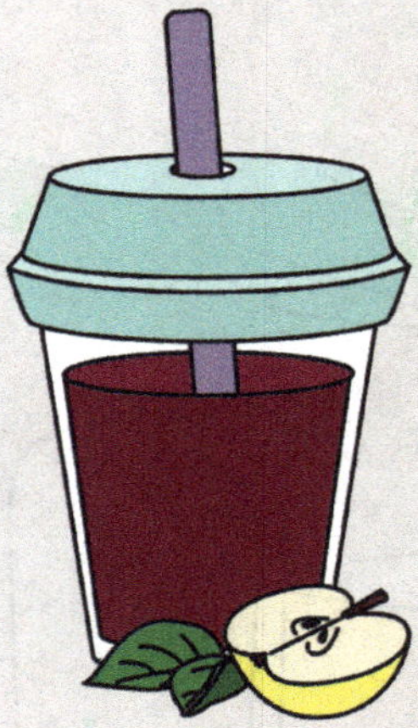

- 1 cup frozen wild blueberries
- $\frac{1}{2}$ cup pomegranate juice
- $\frac{1}{2}$ cup chopped apple (1 small apple)
- $\frac{1}{2}$ cup frozen butternut squash

Calories: ~250

Benefits: Improves memory and brain function with blueberries and pomegranate.

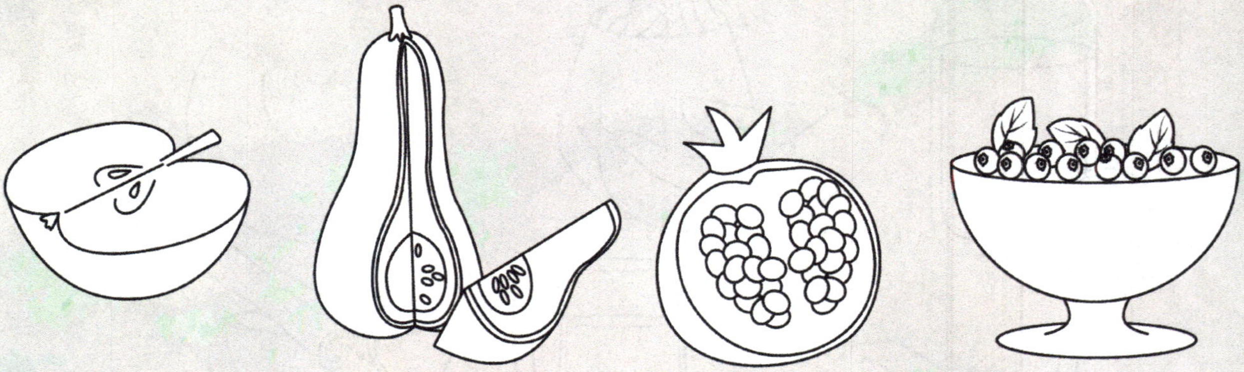

The clarity you feel isn't just physical — it's mental. Focus improves. You don't feel weighed down by digestion, and emotional eating urges reduce.

Running Smooth Smoothie:

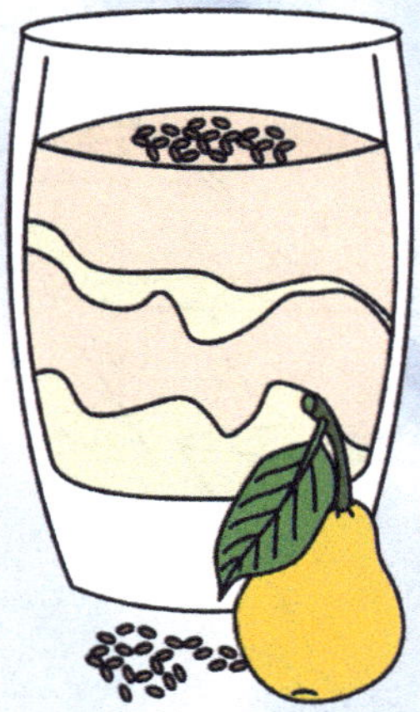

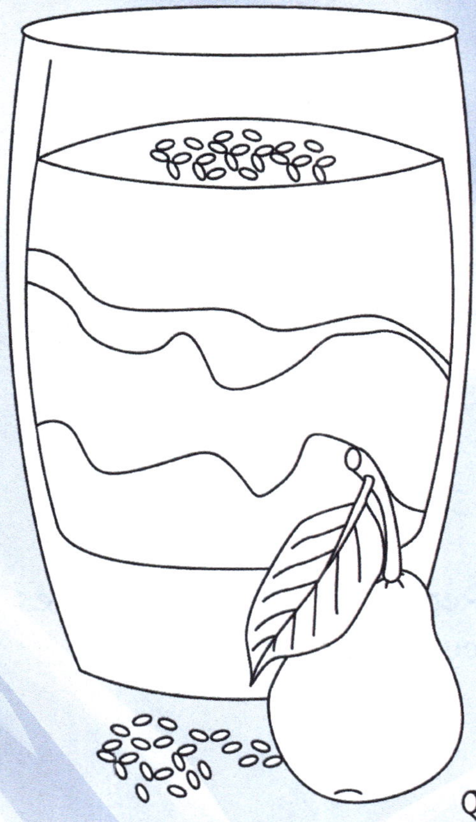

- 1 tsp fresh grated ginger
- $\frac{1}{2}$ cup frozen pears
- 1 pitted date
- $\frac{1}{2}$ cup plain kefir
- 1 tbsp flax seeds

Calories: ~280

Benefits: Supports digestive health with high fiber content.

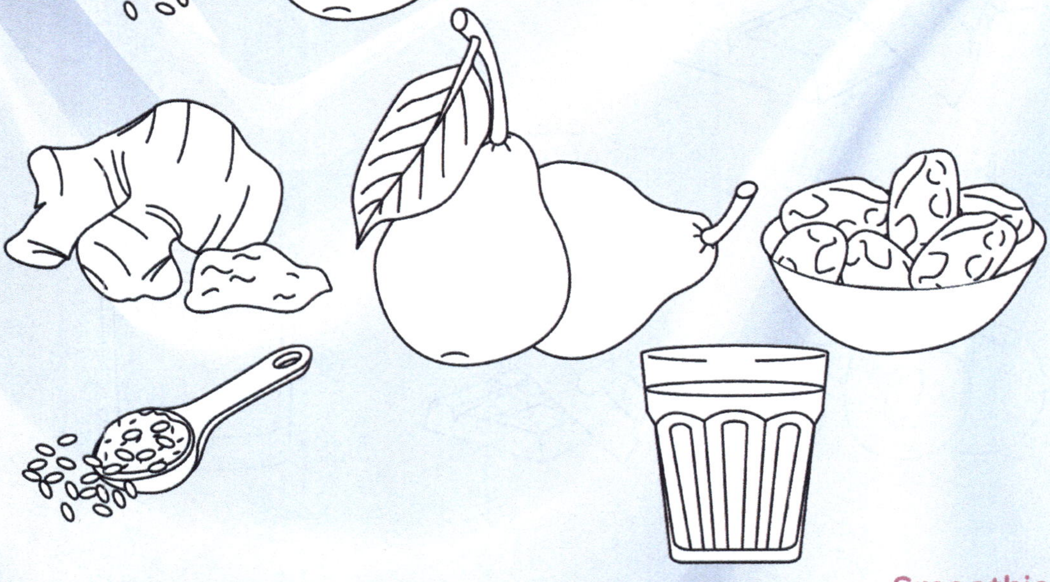

Day 13 - Full Digestive Ease
Smoothie at 10:00 AM and 6:00 PM.

Muscle 911 Smoothie:

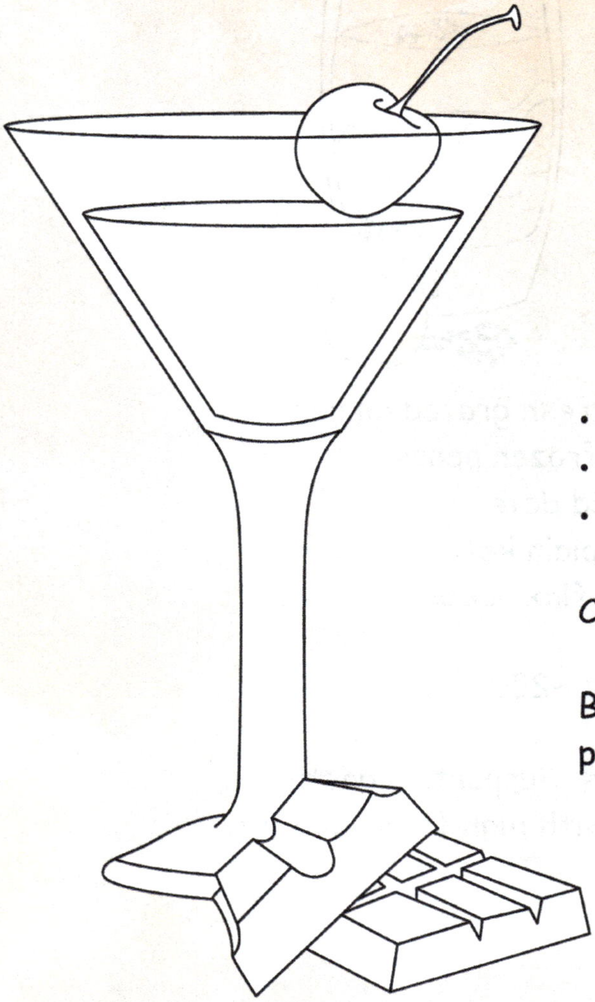

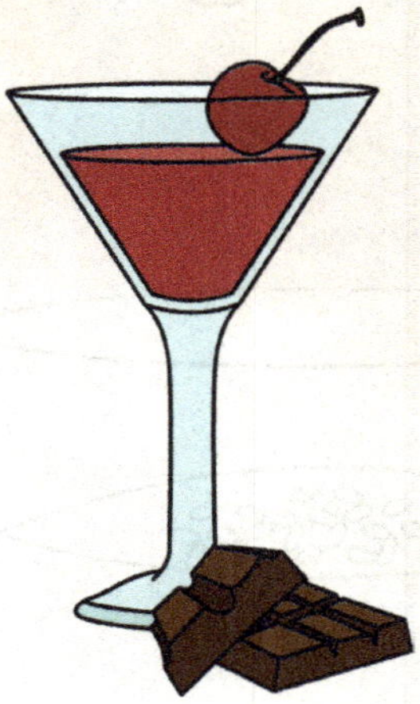

- 1 cup frozen cherries
- 1 cup 2% chocolate milk
- $\frac{1}{4}$ cup tart cherry juice

Calories: ~300

Benefits: Repairs muscles and reduces post-workout inflammation.

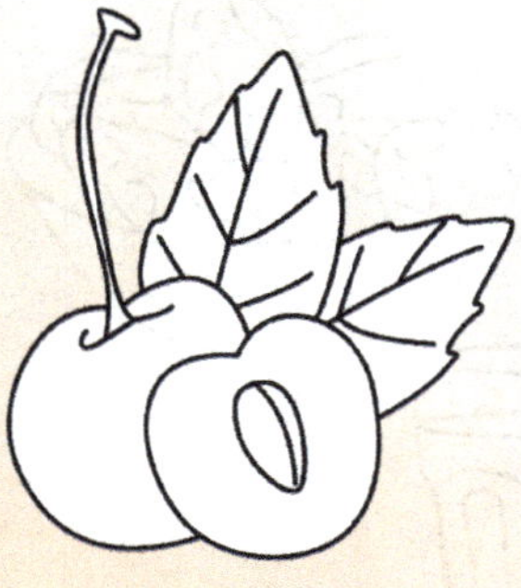

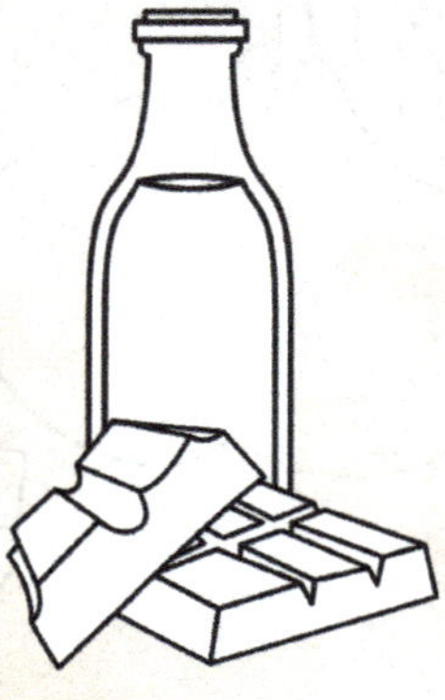

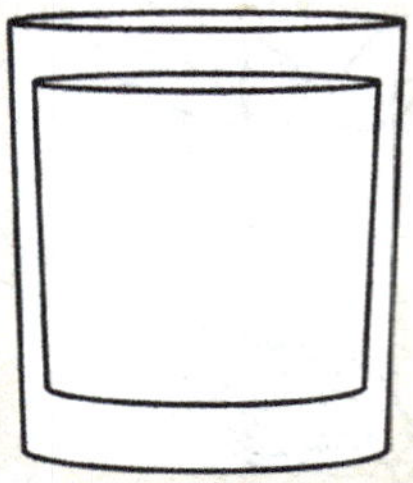

By now, your system works without stress. You may notice better posture, less tension in the stomach area, and smoother elimination. Lightness becomes your new normal.

Bio Beauty Smoothie:

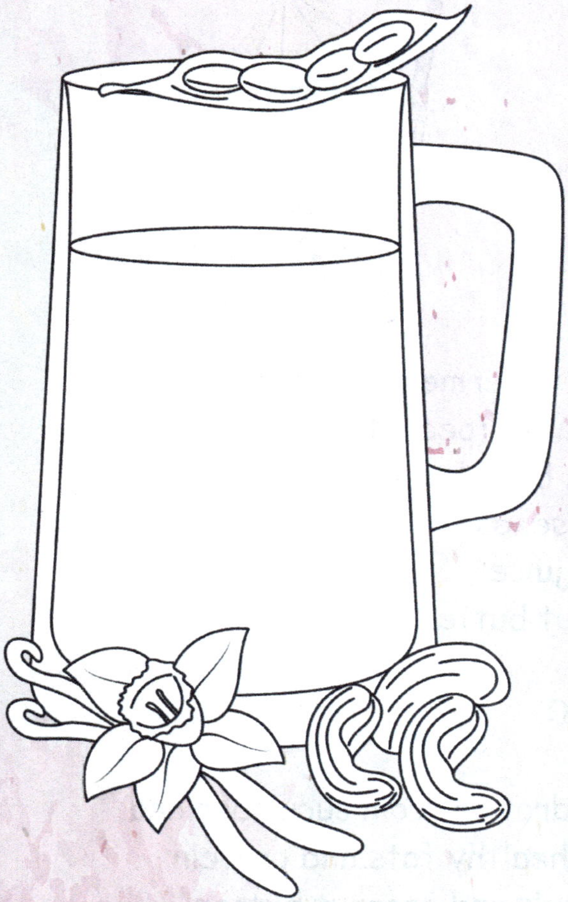

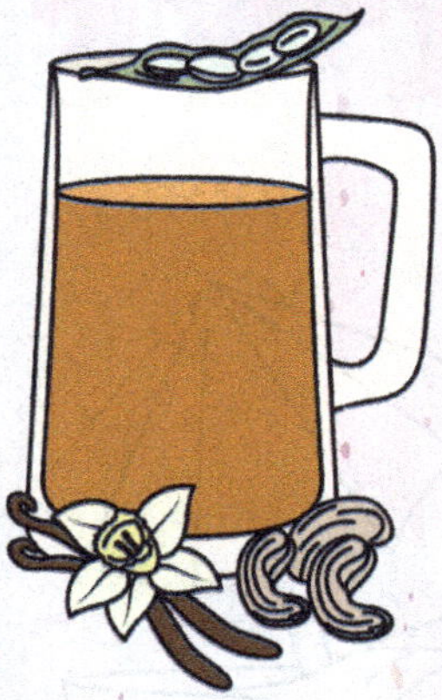

- 1 frozen banana
- $\frac{1}{4}$ cup mashed sweet potatoes
- $\frac{1}{2}$ tsp vanilla extract
- 1 pitted date
- $\frac{1}{4}$ cup cooked white beans
- $\frac{1}{4}$ tsp ground cinnamon
- 1 tsp maple syrup
- $\frac{1}{2}$ cup cashew milk

Calories: ~170

Benefits: Strengthens skin, hair, and nails with biotin-rich ingredients.

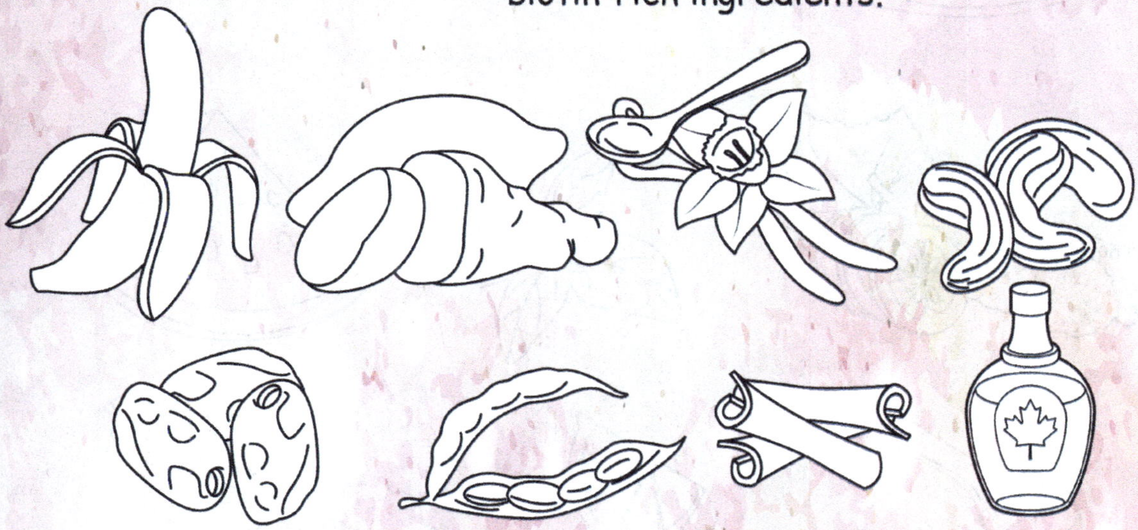

Day 14 – Cellular Refresh

Smoothie at 10:00 AM and 6:00 PM.

Watermelon Cooler:

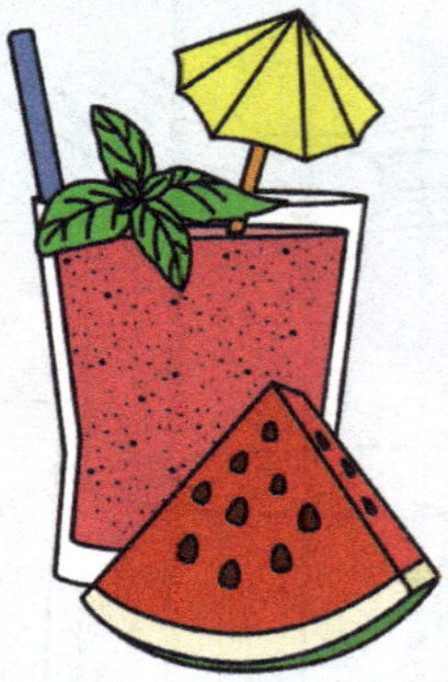

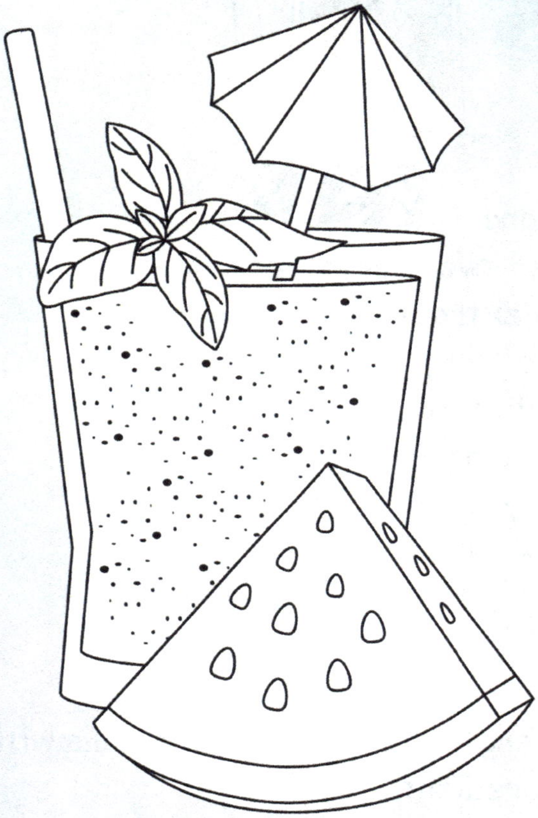

- 1 cup fresh watermelon (cubed)
- $\frac{1}{2}$ cup cucumber (peeled)
- $\frac{1}{4}$ cup fresh basil leaves
- 1 tbsp chia seeds
- 1 tbsp lime juice
- 1 tsp coconut butter

Calories: ~180

Benefits: Hydration from cucumber and watermelon; healthy fats and protein from chia seeds and coconut butter.

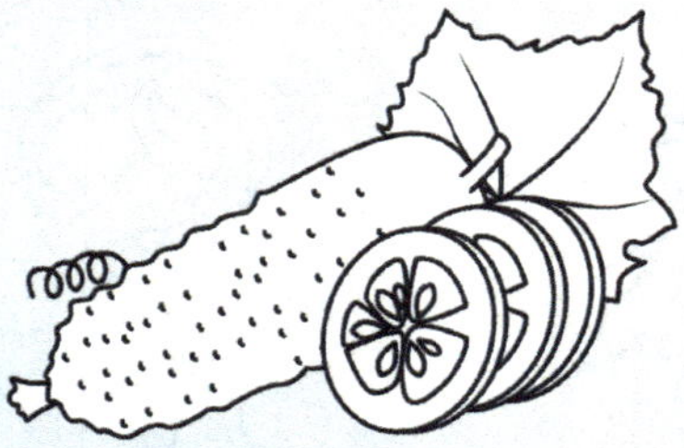

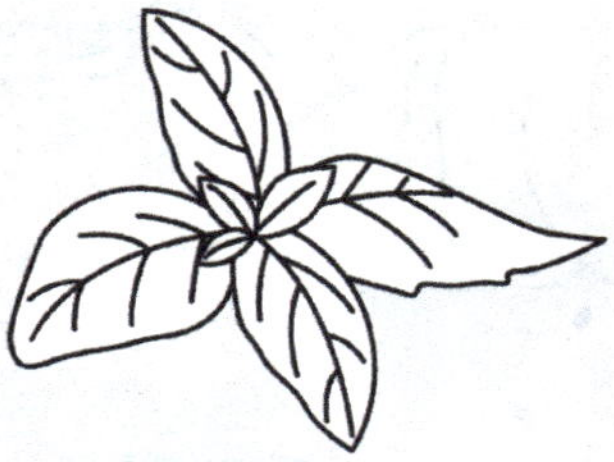

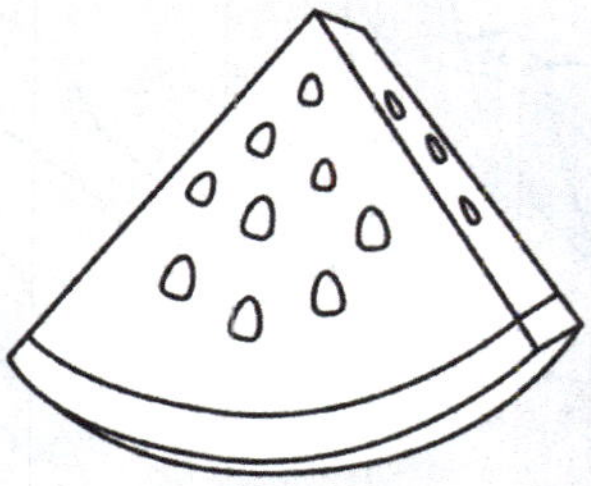

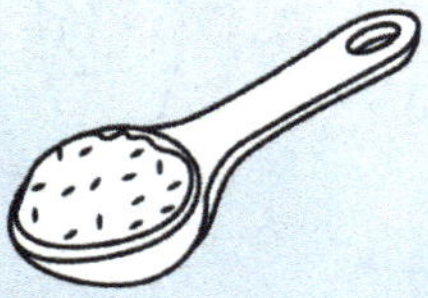

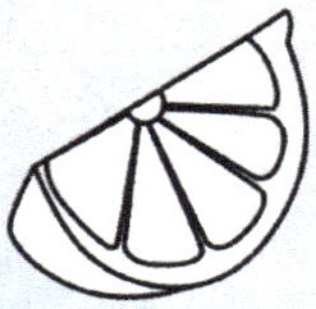

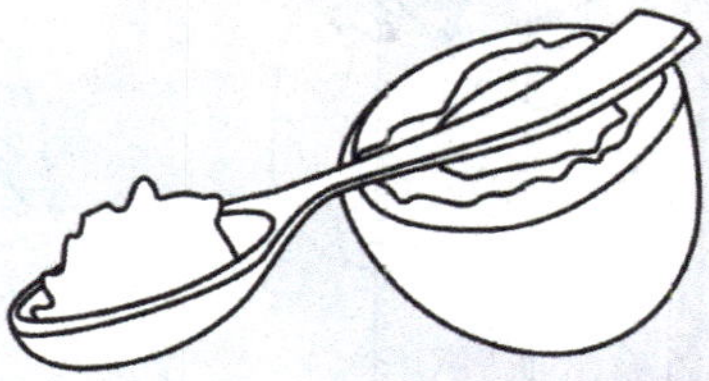

Two weeks in, your body has not only adjusted — it's thriving. Internal inflammation is lower, digestion is balanced, and your stomach feels clean, strong, and calm.

Lemon Blueberry Smoothie:

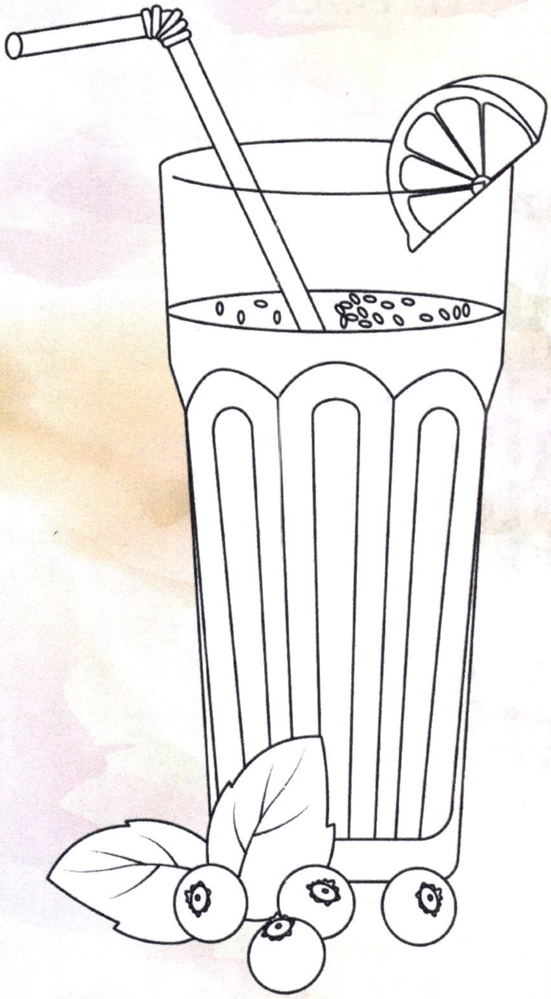

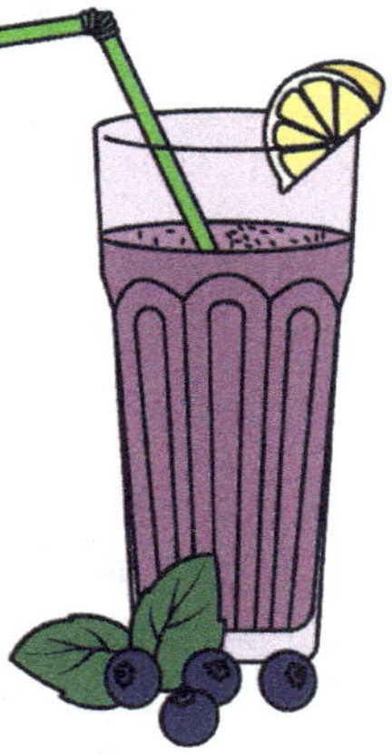

- $\frac{1}{2}$ cup frozen cauliflower
- $\frac{1}{2}$ cup blueberries
- 1 tbsp almond butter
- 1 tbsp flaxseed meal
- 1 tbsp lemon juice

Calories: ~200

Benefits: Antioxidant-rich, promotes digestion; creamy texture suitable for a smoothie bowl.

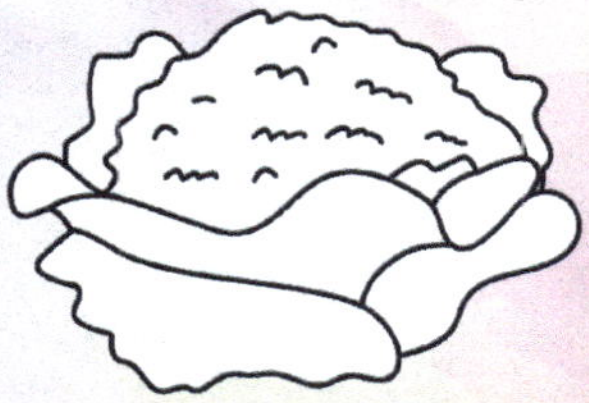

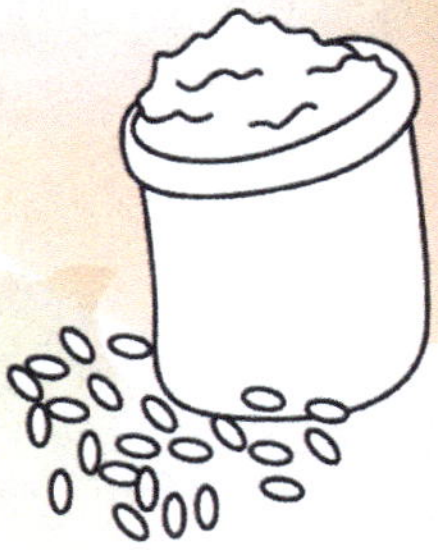

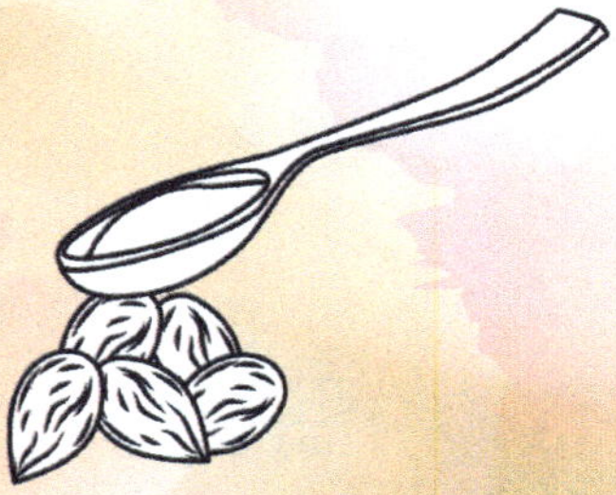

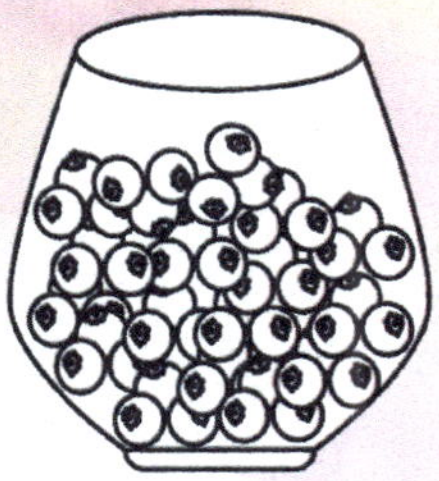

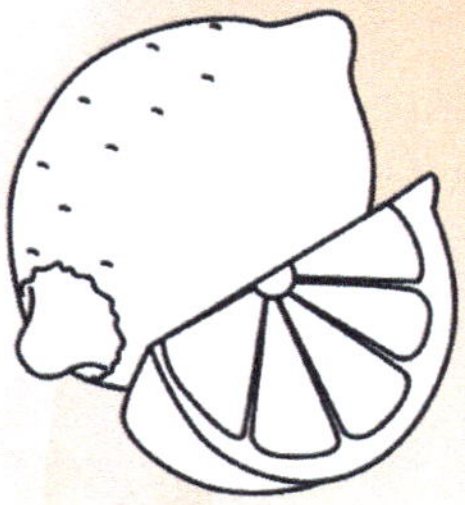

Thank you so much for reading this book!

We'd Love to hear from You

Review on Amazon

Scan me

Weekly Wellness Check-In

Weight This Week ____________________

____

____

Favorite Smoothie ____________________

____

____

Mood This Week ____________________

____

____

Notes ____________________

____

Day 15 – Switching to a Hearty Morning

Hearty breakfast; smoothies for lunch and dinner.

Chocolate Cherry Pie Smoothie:

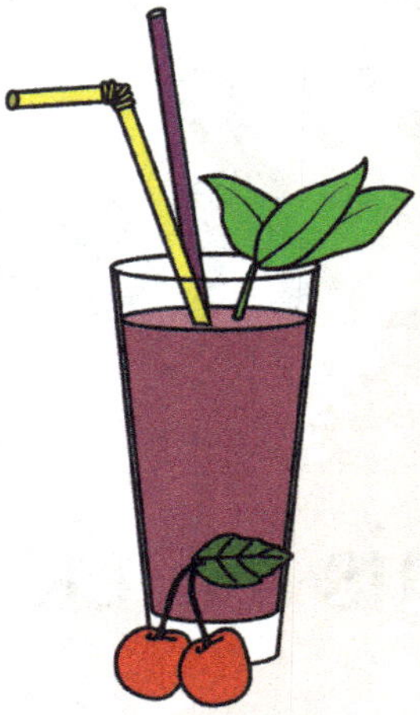

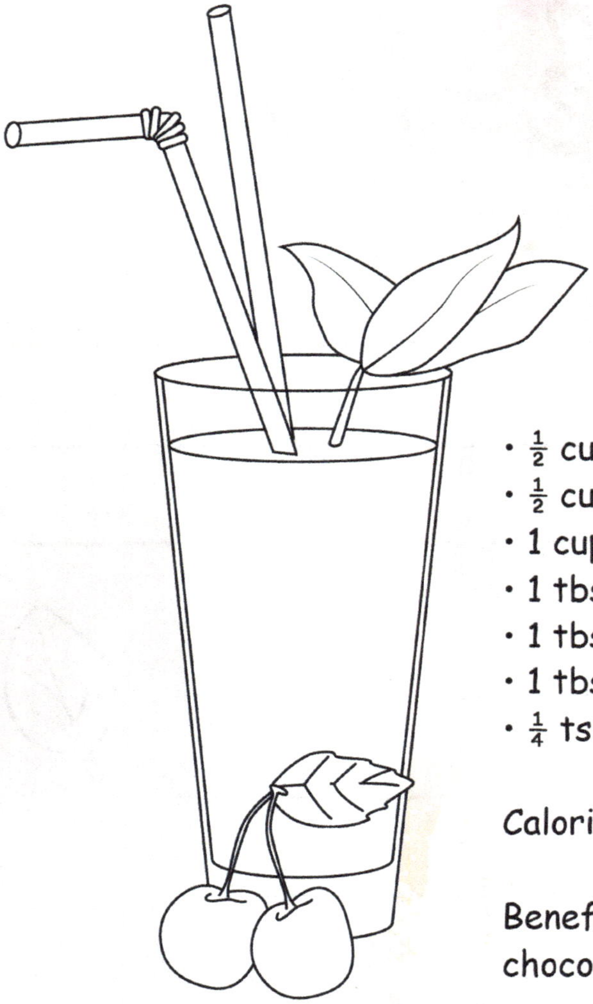

- $\frac{1}{2}$ cup frozen cherries
- $\frac{1}{2}$ cup cucumber (peeled)
- 1 cup spinach
- 1 tbsp hemp seeds
- 1 tbsp cacao powder
- 1 tbsp cashew butter
- $\frac{1}{4}$ tsp cinnamon

Calories: ~280

Benefits: Packed with protein and healthy fats; chocolatey, dessert-like taste.

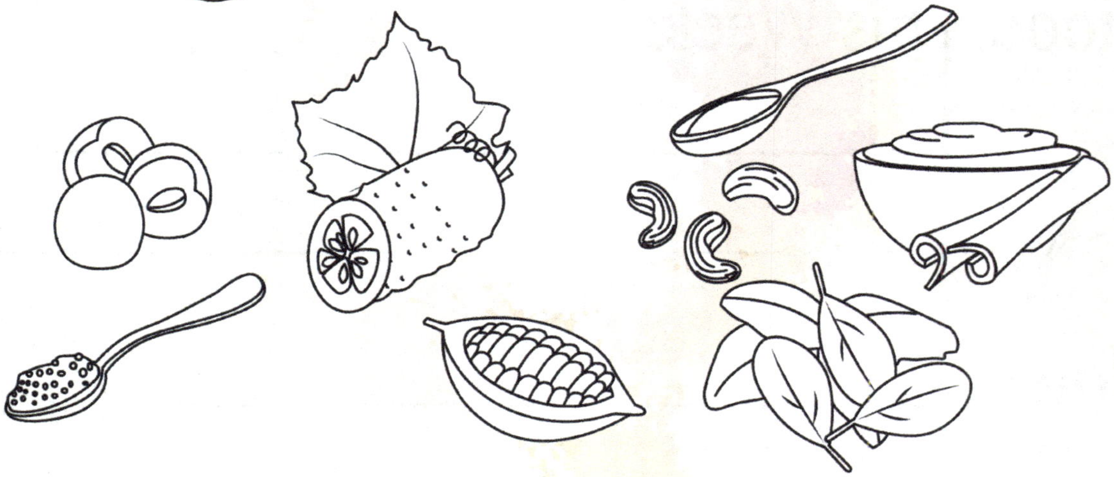

Your body gets energy early in the day, which reduces evening hunger. Smoothies during the day and evening keep your stomach light and help you ease into this new rhythm.

Peanut Butter & Greens Smoothie:

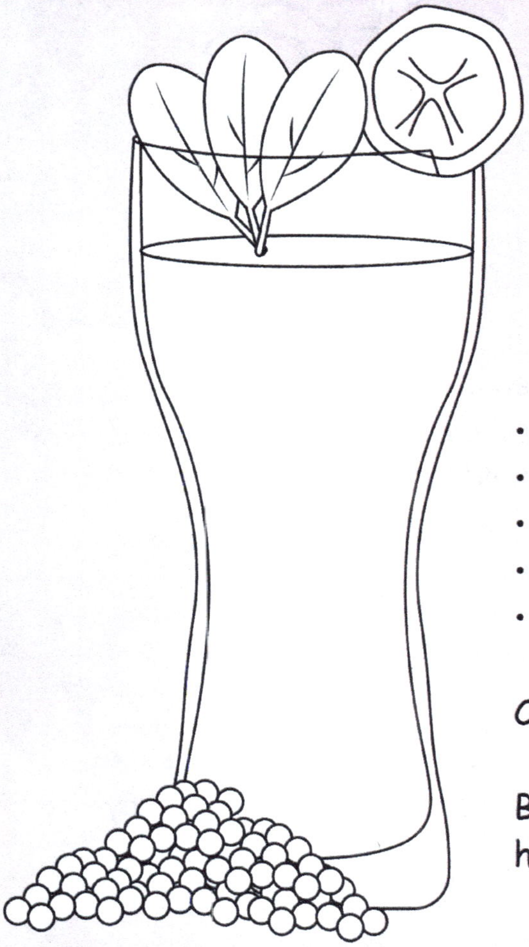

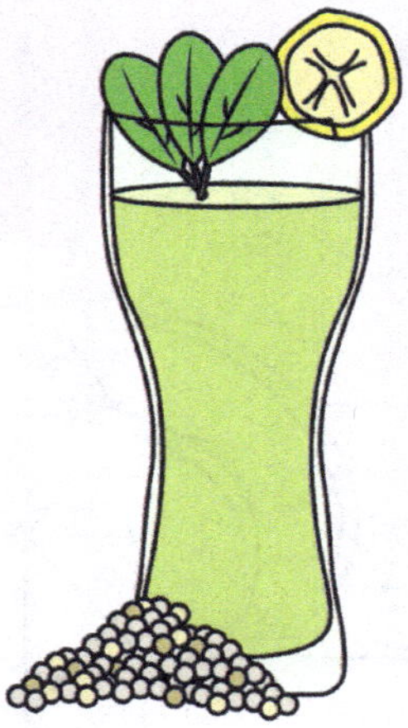

- 1 cup spinach
- $\frac{1}{2}$ cup zucchini (chopped)
- $\frac{1}{2}$ frozen banana
- 1 tbsp peanut butter
- 2 tbsp quinoa flakes

Calories: ~250

Benefits: Creamy texture with hydration; peanut buttery flavor.

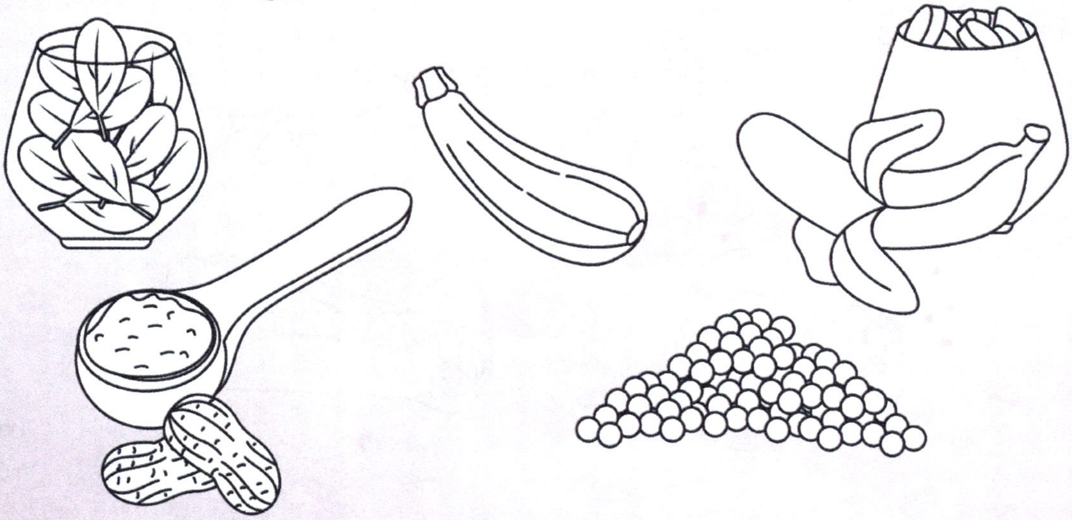

Day 16 – Boosted Metabolism

Hearty breakfast; smoothies for lunch and dinner.

Creamy Apple Pie Smoothie:

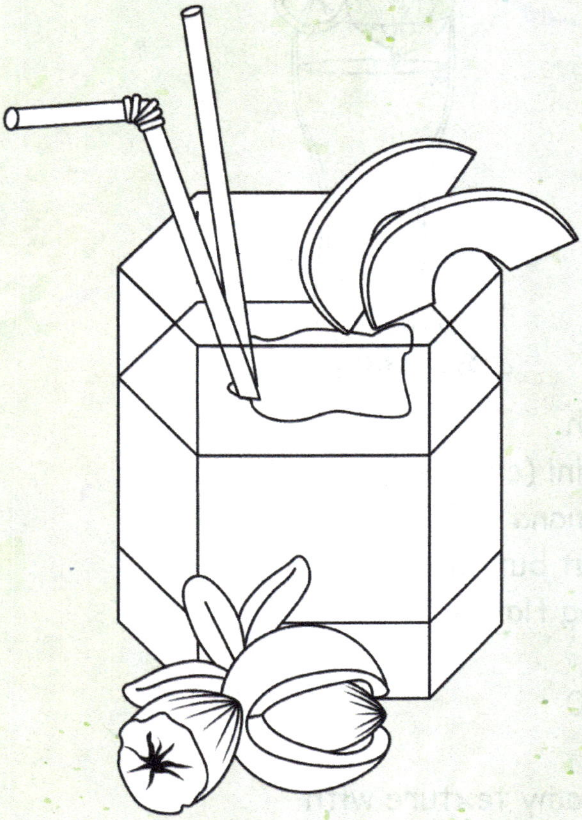

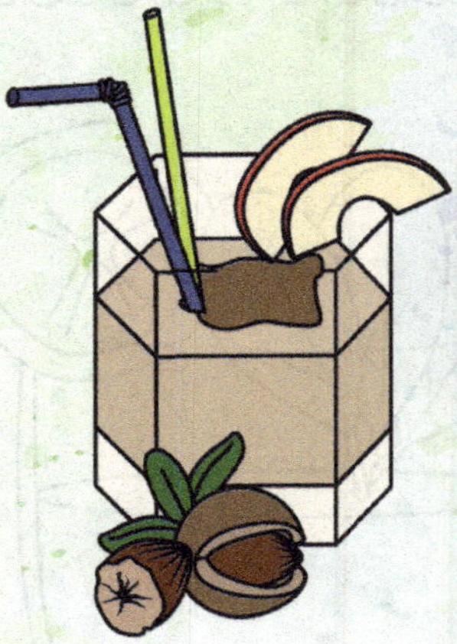

- 1 cup frozen apples
- $\frac{1}{4}$ cup rolled oats
- 1 tbsp almond butter
- $\frac{1}{2}$ tsp cinnamon
- $\frac{1}{4}$ tsp nutmeg

Calories: ~220

Benefits: Autumn-inspired, tastes like apple pie; refreshing start to the day.

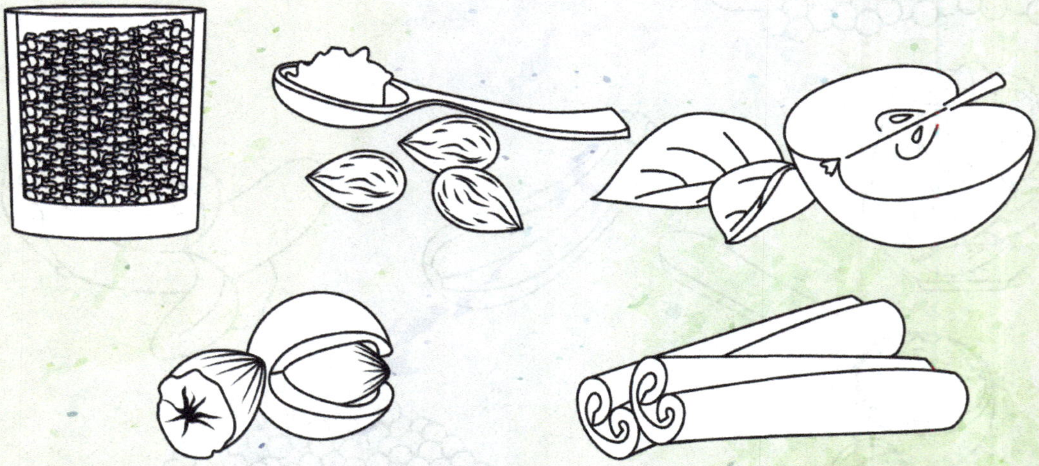

A full breakfast kick-starts your metabolism for the day. Smoothies maintain balance without overeating. Weight starts to stabilize or naturally decrease.

Peanut Butter Chocolate Smoothie: :

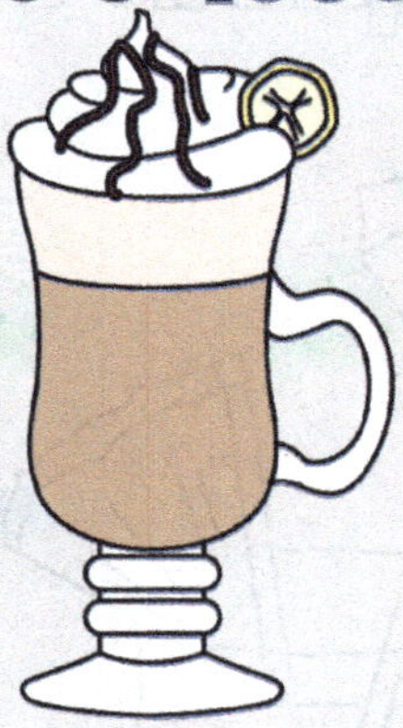

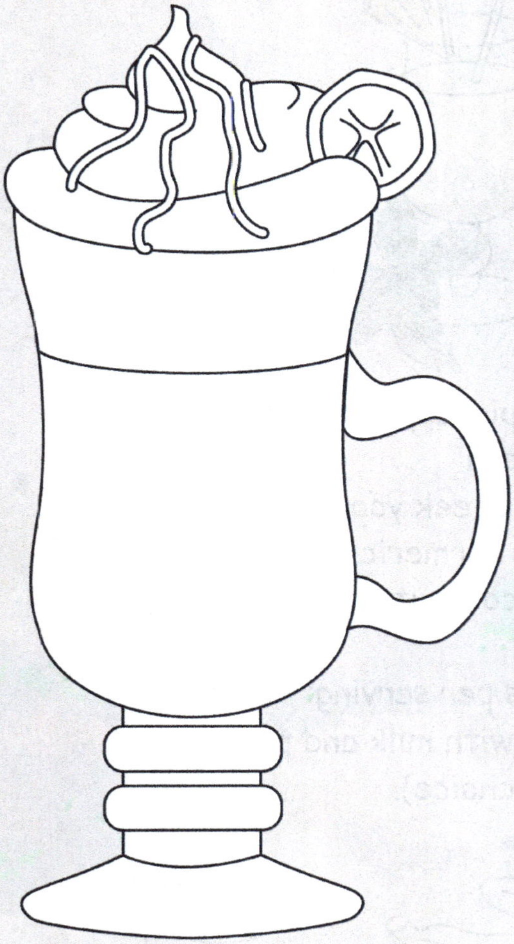

- 1 ripe banana: Natural sweetness + potassium for muscle function.
- 2 tbsp peanut butter: Plant-based protein + heart-healthy fats.
- 1 tbsp unsweetened cocoa powder: Antioxidant-rich with mood-boosting magnesium.
- 1 cup milk: Dairy or plant-based for creaminess + calcium.

Ice cubes: For a thick, frosty texture.

Calories per serving: ~230 (varies with milk and peanut butter choice).

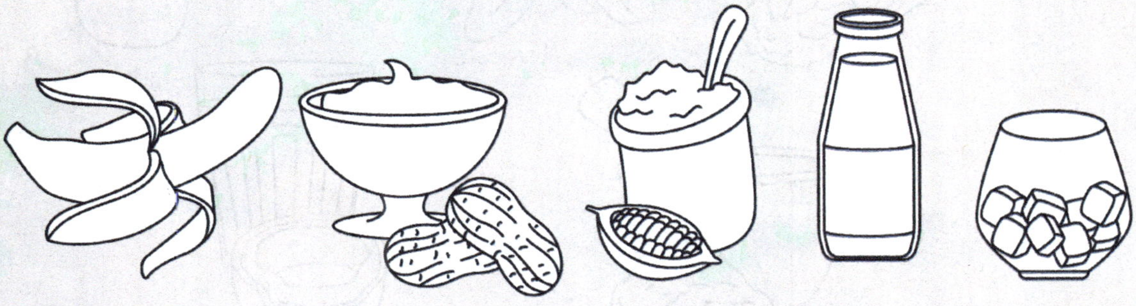

Day 17 – Stomach Comfort

Hearty breakfast; smoothies for lunch and dinner.

Tropical Slim Down Smoothie:

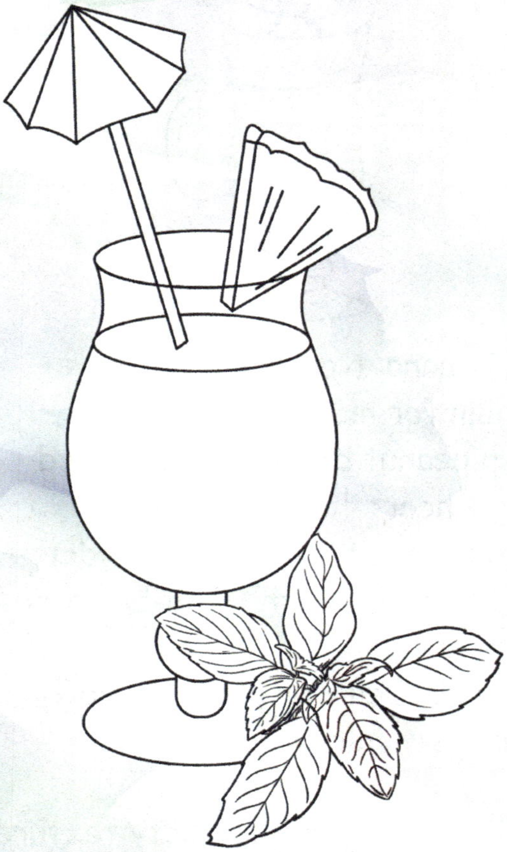

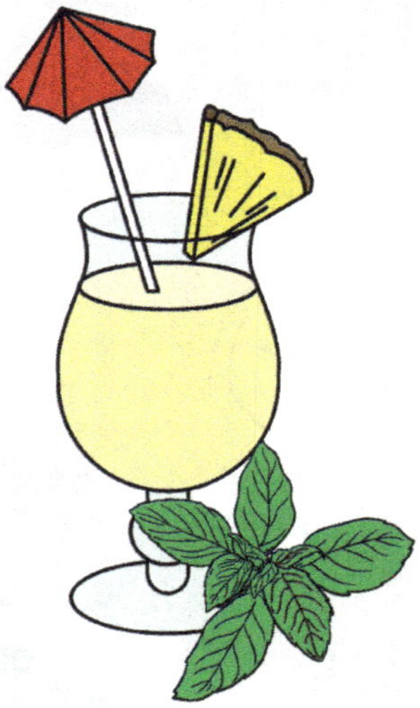

- 1 cup pineapple chunks
- ½ banana
- ½ cup Greek yogurt
- 1 tbsp turmeric
- 1 cup coconut milk

Calories per serving: ~230 (varies with milk and peanut butter choice).

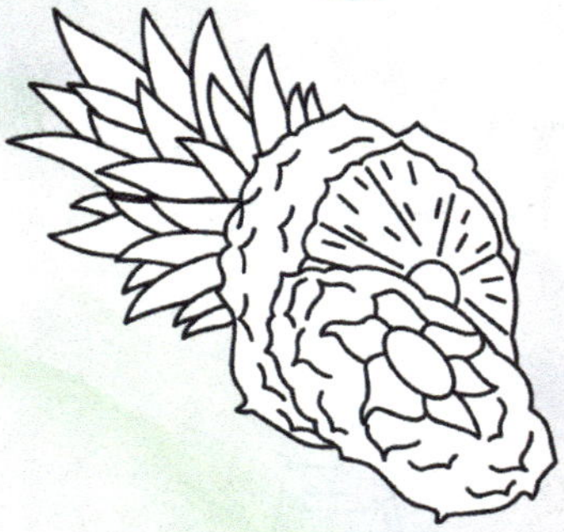

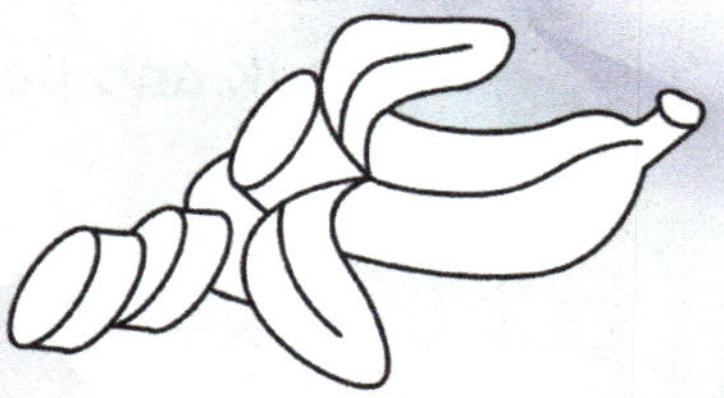

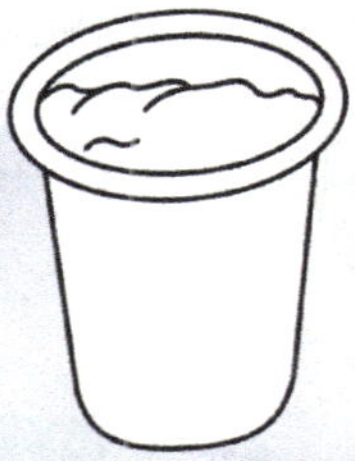

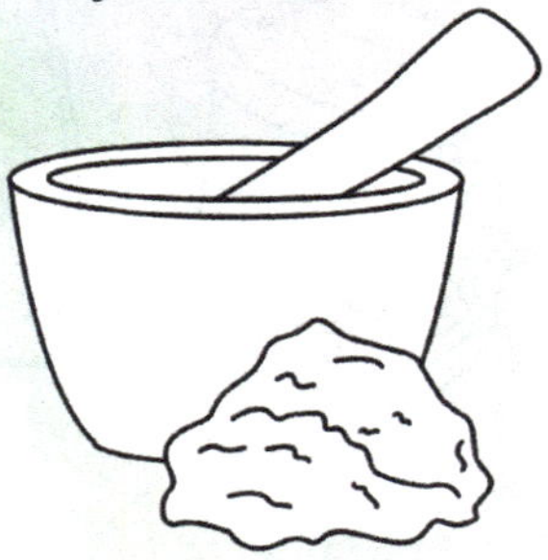

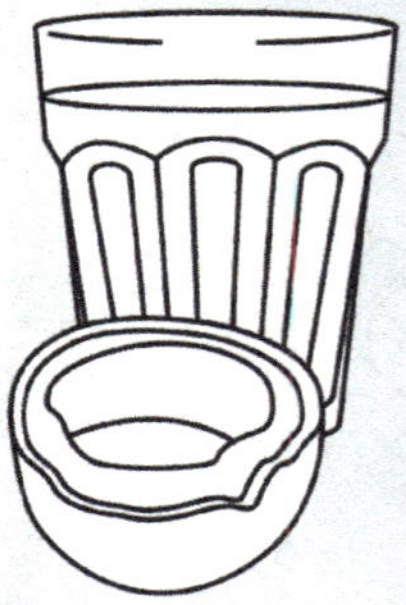

You fuel up in the morning for productivity, while your stomach rests later in the day. Digestion becomes calm and effortless, without heaviness.

Berry Fat Burner Smoothie:

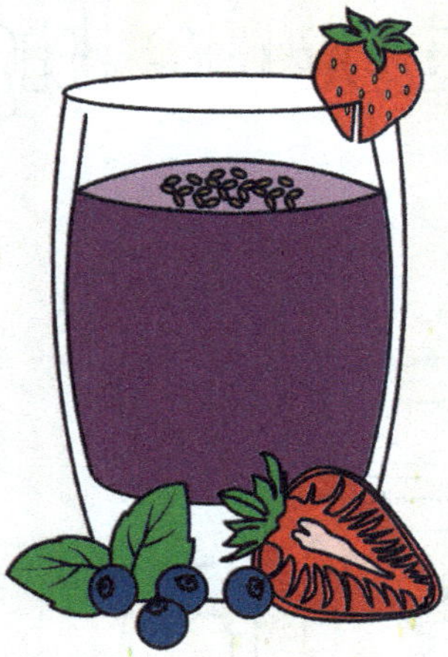

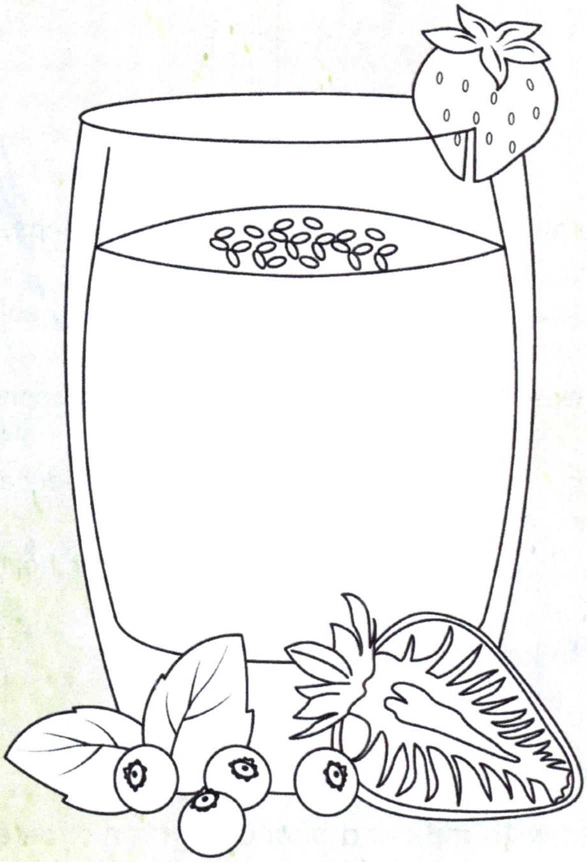

- $\frac{1}{2}$ cup frozen blueberries
- $\frac{1}{2}$ cup fresh or frozen strawberries
- 1 tbsp flaxseeds
- 1 cup unsweetened almond milk
- $\frac{1}{2}$ ripe banana

Calories per serving: ~230 (varies with milk and peanut butter choice).

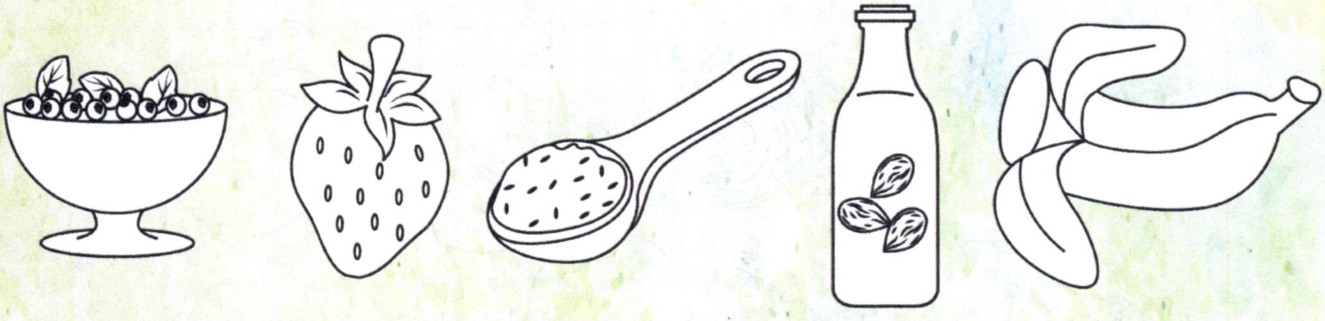

Day 18 - More Nutrients, Less Stress

Hearty breakfast; smoothies for lunch and dinner.

Apple and Black Grape Smoothie Ingredients (Serves 1):

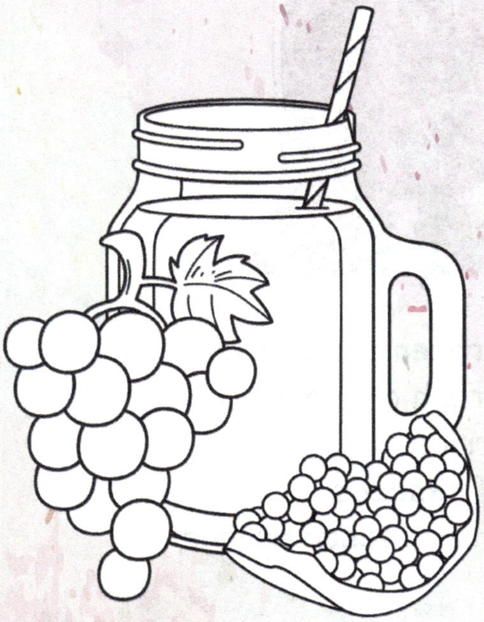

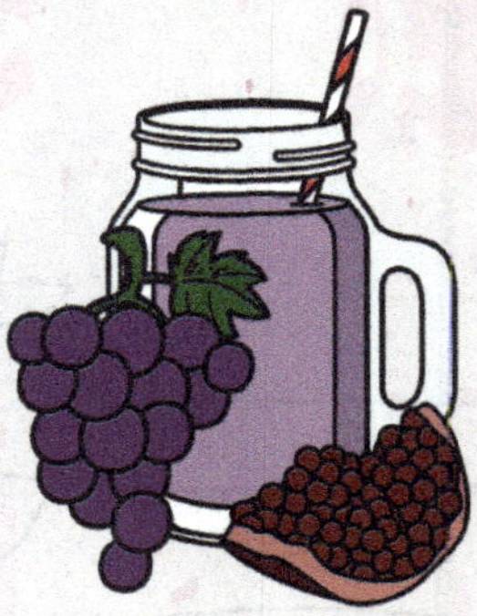

- 3 tbsp old-fashioned rolled oats: Slow-release carbs for lasting energy.
- 10 soaked cashew nuts: Creamy texture + healthy fats.
- $\frac{3}{4}$ cup water: Hydrating base (swap with coconut water for electrolytes).
- 1 rough-chopped apple: Fiber-rich with quercetin for immunity.
- 1 tbsp flax seeds: Omega-3s + lignans for hormone balance.
- 1 tbsp chia seeds: Fiber + protein to keep you full.
- 1 cup seedless black grapes: Antioxidant-packed resveratrol.

Pomegranate seeds (garnish): Adds crunch + extra antioxidants.

Calories per serving: ~230 (varies with milk and peanut butter choice).

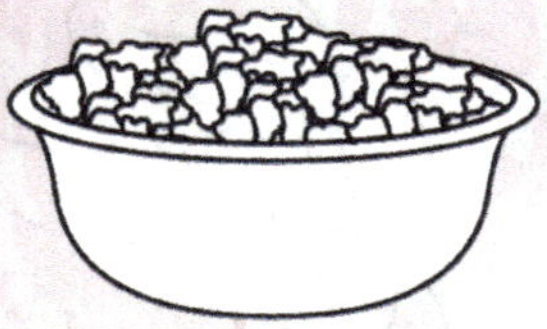
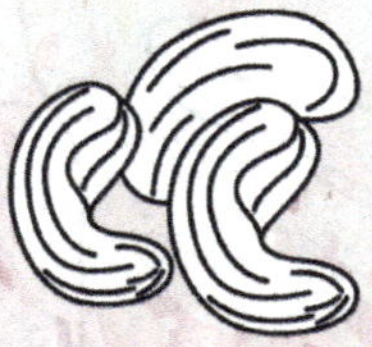
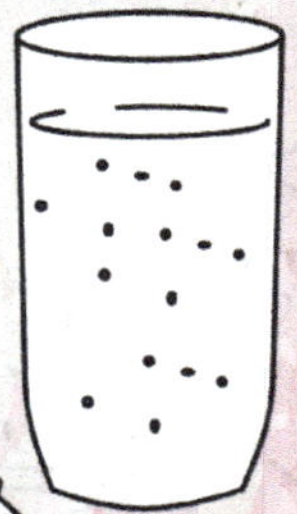
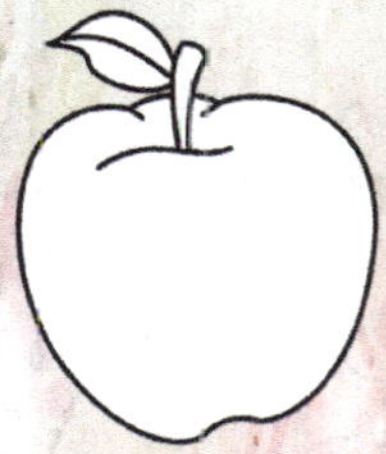
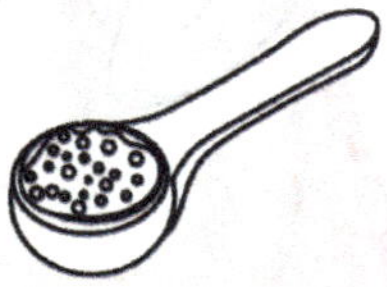
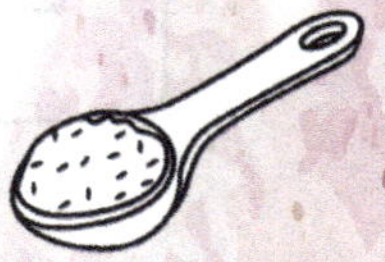
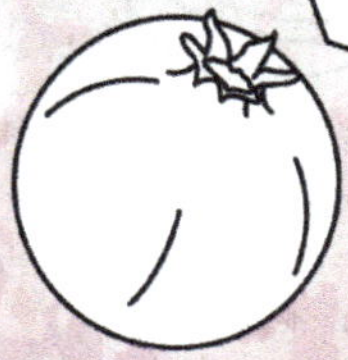

Smoothies provide antioxidants and support immunity. No more stress around eating or calorie counting — you know your body is getting what it needs.

Coffee Breakfast Smoothie

Ingredients (Serves 1):

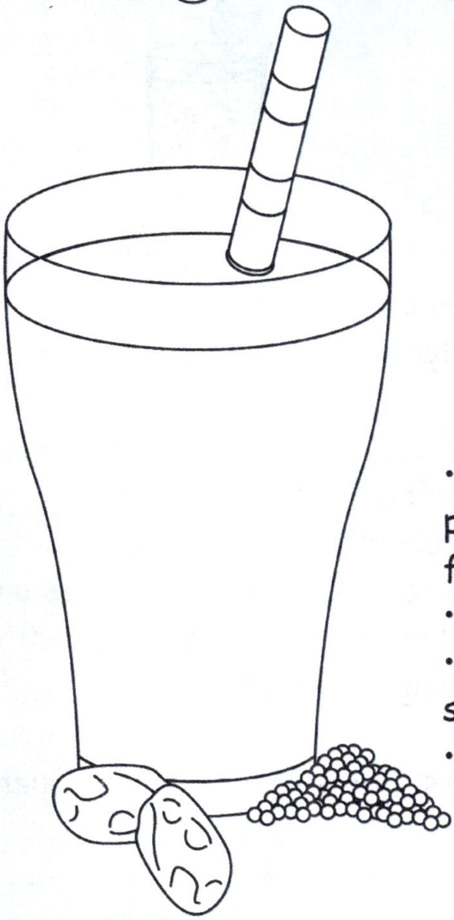

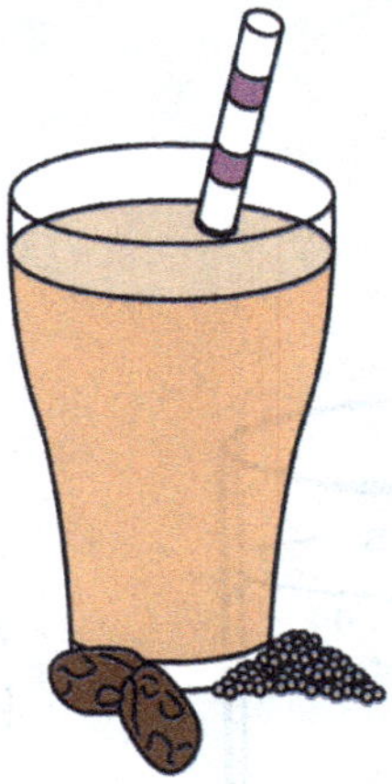

- 1 large ripe banana (previously peeled, sliced and frozen // more for a sweeter smoothie)
- 1 cup fresh orange juice
- 1/2 Tbsp fresh ginger (peeled // 1 small knob yields ~1/2 Tbsp)
- 1/2 cup carrot juice

Total Number of Calories
~200-250 per serving (varies with milk, yogurt type, and added sweeteners).

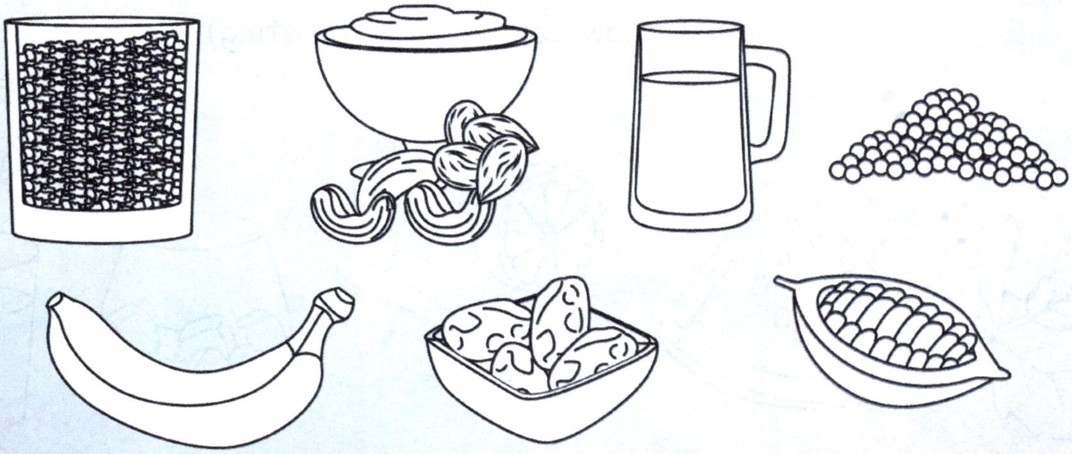

Day 19 - Stable Energy, No Slumps
Hearty breakfast; smoothies for lunch and dinner.

Watermelon Mint Smoothie

Ingredients (Serves 2):

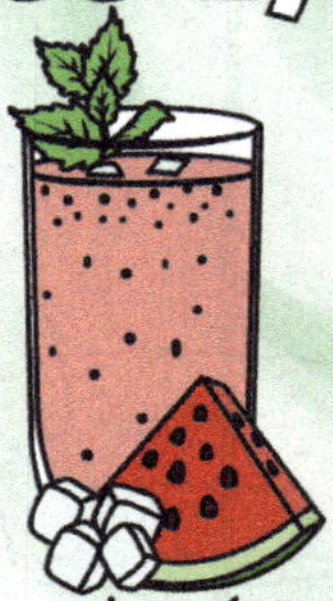

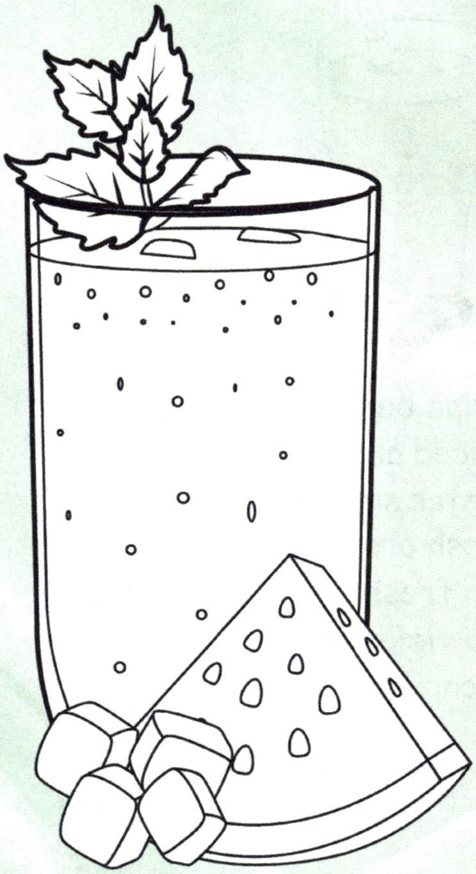

• 1 cup diced watermelon (seedless): 92% water + lycopene for hydration and skin health.
• ½ cup fresh mint leaves: Aids digestion + adds refreshing brightness.
• ½ cup coconut water: Natural electrolytes (potassium + magnesium).
• 1 tbsp lime juice: Vitamin C boost + detoxifying enzymes.

Ice cubes: For a frosty, thirst-quenching texture.

Calories per serving: ~45 (naturally low-calorie and hydrating).

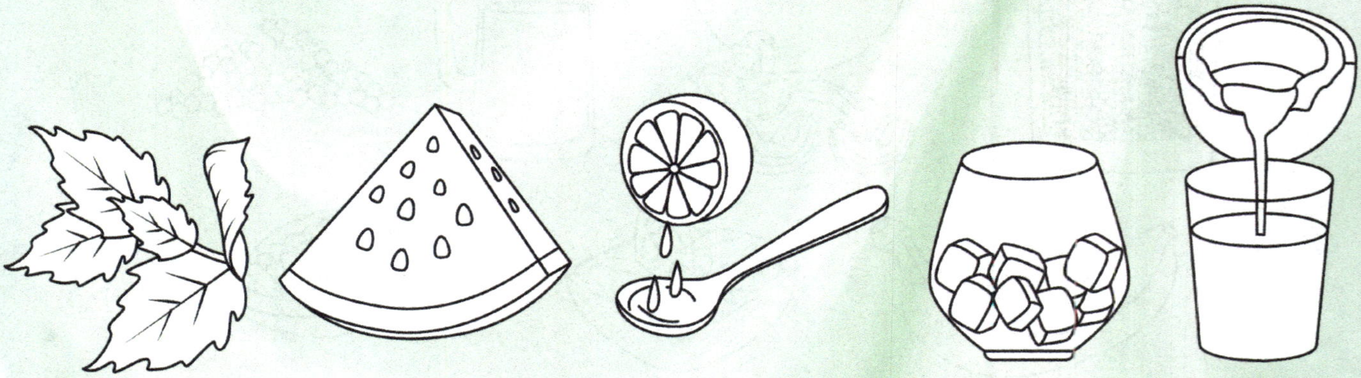

No energy crashes. Smoothies digest easily and leave energy for work, movement, or rest. The stomach stays calm all the way through bedtime.

Peach Mango Smoothie Ingredients (Serves 2):

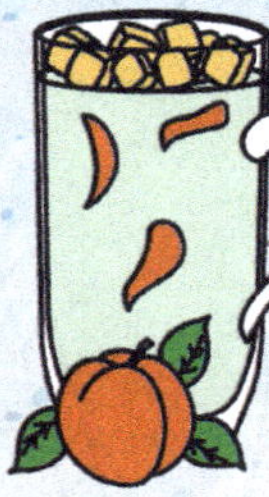

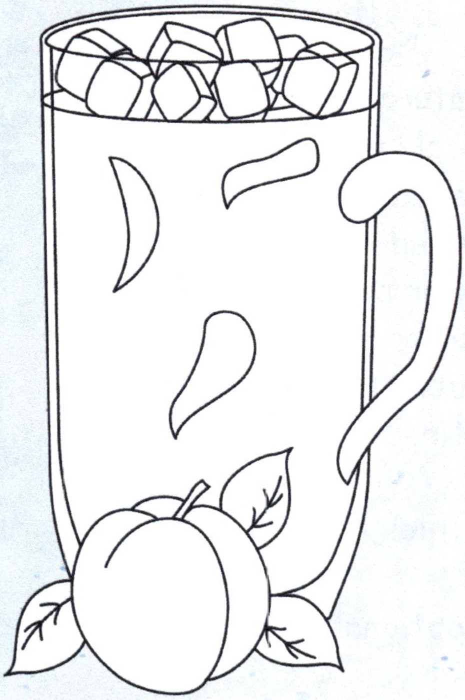

- 1 cup frozen peach slices: Rich in vitamins A + C for glowing skin.
- 1 cup frozen mango chunks: Tropical sweetness + digestive enzymes.
- ½ cup Greek yogurt: Probiotics + 12g protein (use coconut yogurt for vegan).
- ½ cup orange juice: Freshly squeezed for vitamin C + zesty brightness.

Ice cubes: For a frosty, refreshing texture.

Calories per serving: ~140 (varies with yogurt and juice choices).

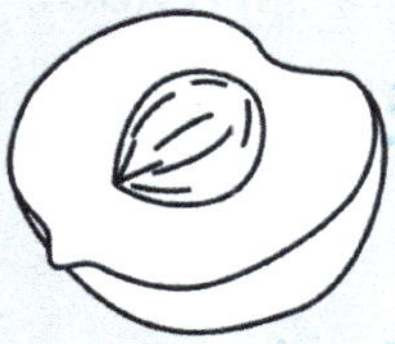

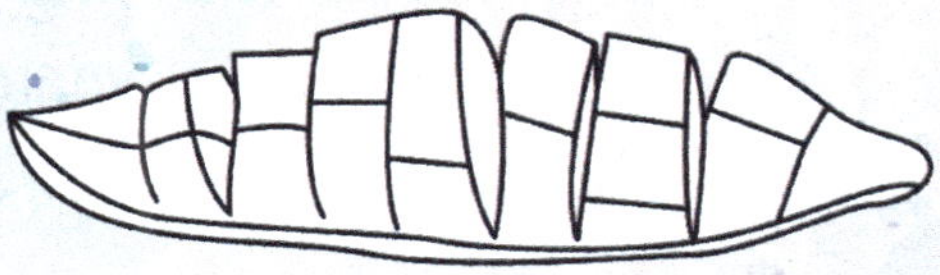

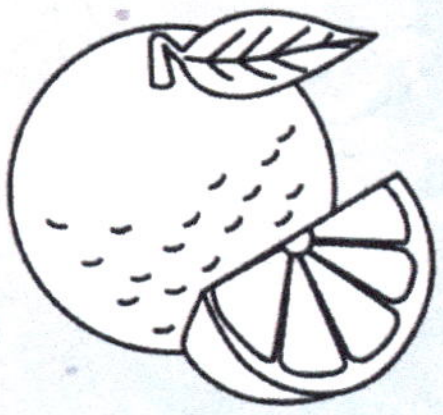

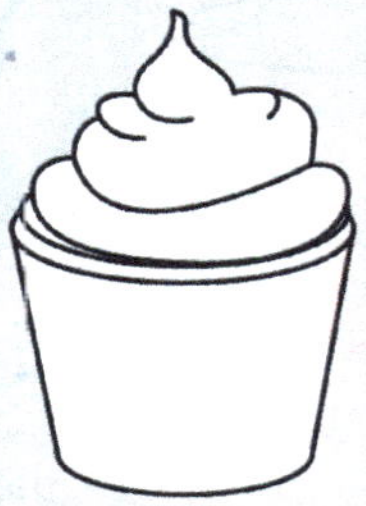

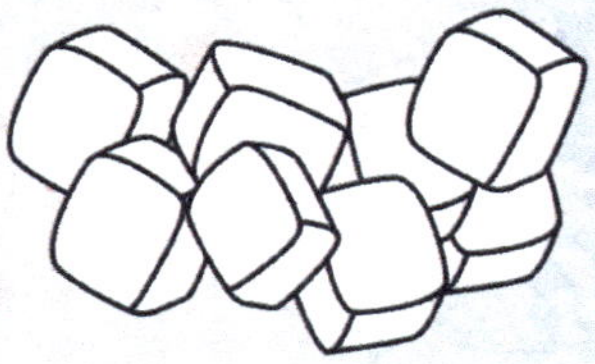

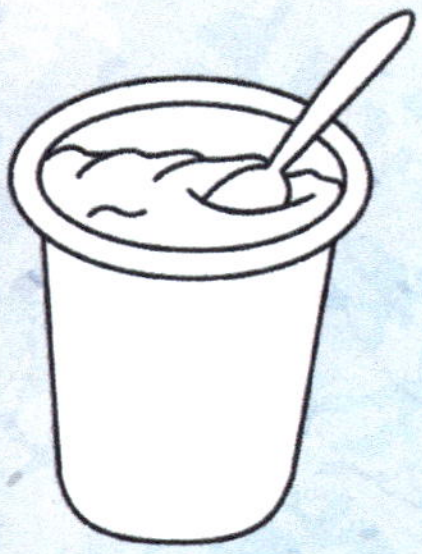

Day 20 - Confident Body

Hearty breakfast; smoothies for lunch and dinner.

Chocolate Banana Smoothie

Ingredients (Serves 2):

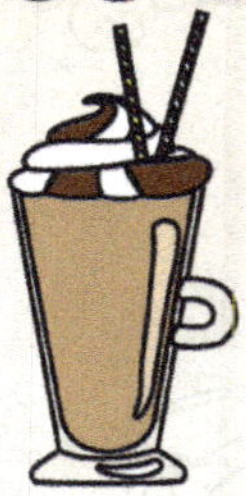

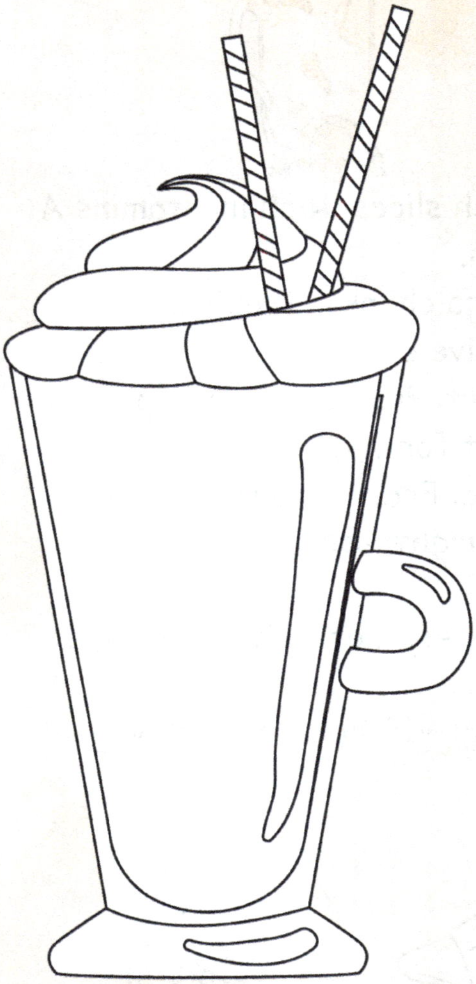

- 1 ripe banana: Natural sweetness + potassium for muscle recovery.
- 2 tbsp unsweetened cocoa powder: Rich in flavonoids and magnesium.
- 1 cup milk: Dairy or plant-based for creaminess + calcium.
- 1 tbsp peanut butter: Healthy fats + plant-based protein.

Ice cubes: For a thick, frosty texture.

Whipped cream (optional): Adds a decadent finish.

Calories per serving: ~187 (without whipped cream; varies with milk choice).

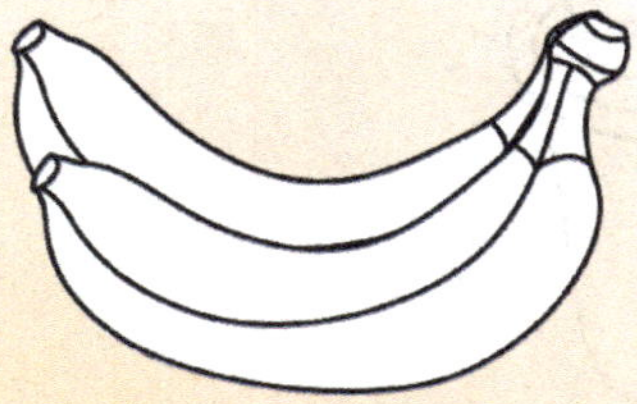

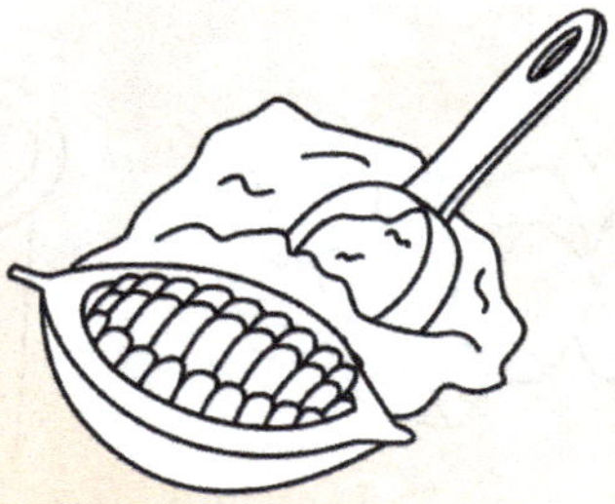

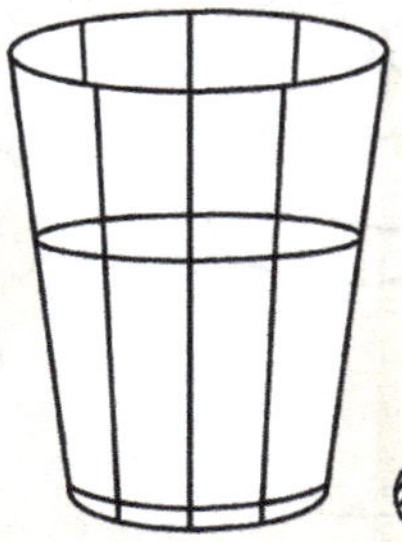

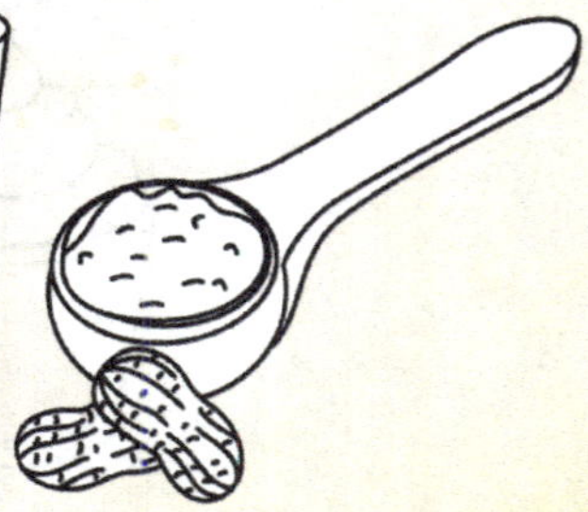

No bloating or heaviness — just lightness and clarity. Digestion is steady, skin looks fresher. You feel grounded and strong from the morning onward.

Kiwi Strawberry Smoothie Ingredients (Serves 2):

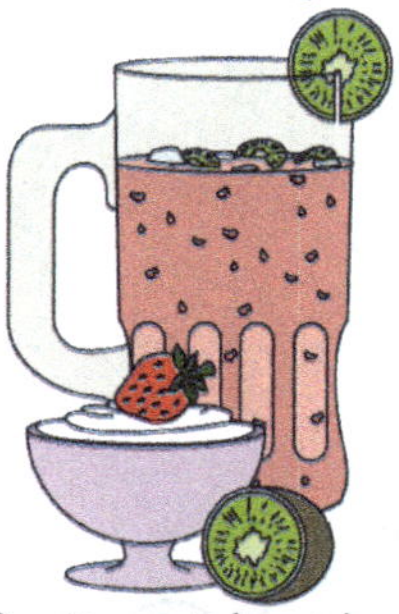

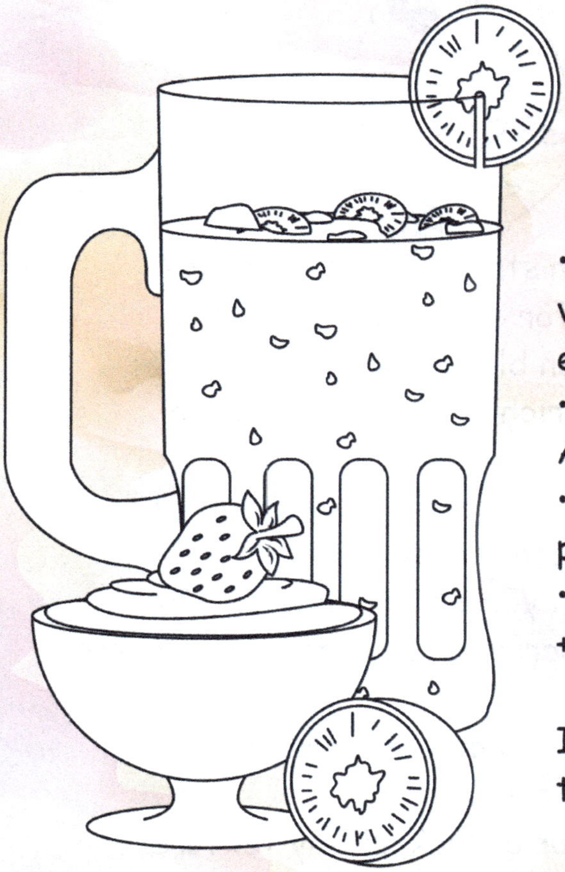

• 2 ripe kiwis (peeled): Double the vitamin C of oranges + digestive enzymes.
• 1 cup frozen strawberries: Antioxidant-rich for glowing skin.
• ½ cup Greek yogurt: Probiotics + 10g protein (use coconut yogurt for vegan).
• ½ cup coconut water: Natural hydration + potassium.

Ice cubes: For a frosty, thirst-quenching texture.

Calories per serving: ~135 (varies with yogurt choice).

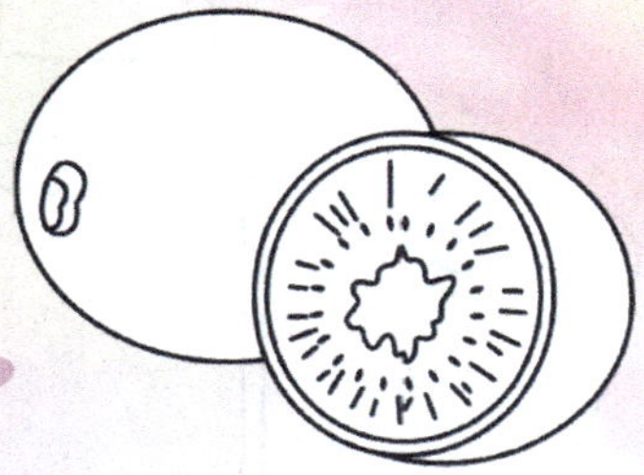
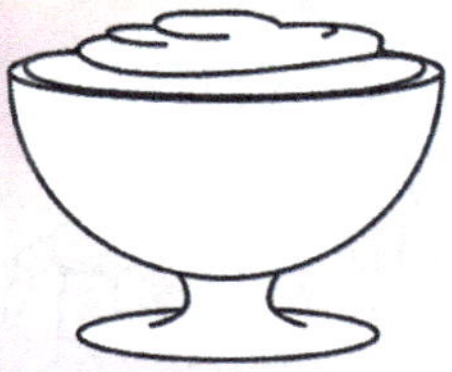

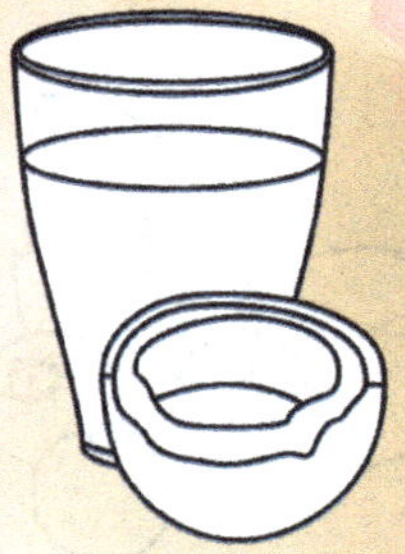

Day 21 – Balanced System

Hearty breakfast; smoothies for lunch and dinner.

Berry Blast Smoothie Ingredients (Serves 2):

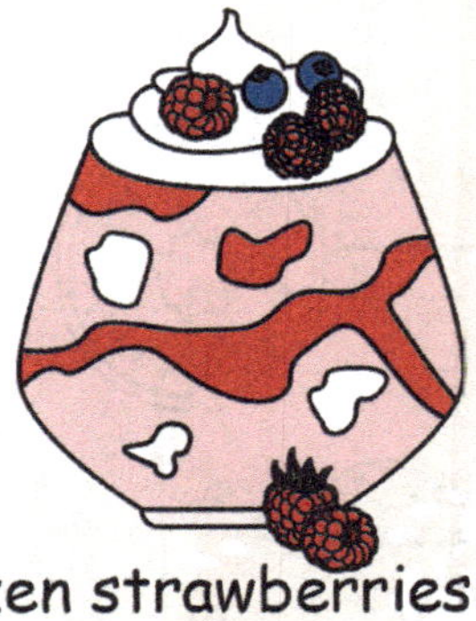

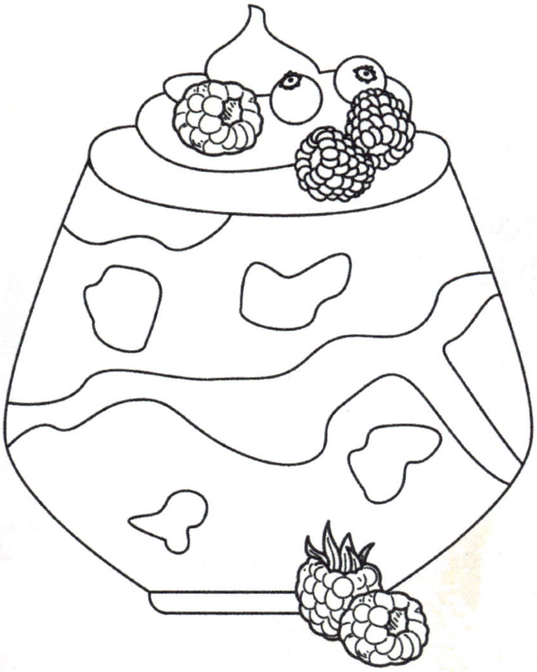

- $\frac{1}{2}$ cup frozen strawberries: Vitamin C powerhouse for collagen synthesis.
- $\frac{1}{2}$ cup frozen blueberries: Antioxidant-rich with brain-boosting anthocyanins.
- $\frac{1}{2}$ cup frozen raspberries: High in fiber + anti-inflammatory ellagic acid.
- $\frac{1}{2}$ cup Greek yogurt: Probiotics + 11g protein per serving (use almond yogurt for vegan).

$\frac{1}{2}$ cup milk: Dairy or plant-based for creaminess + calcium.

Ice cubes: For a thick, slushy texture.

Whipped cream (optional): Adds indulgent flair.

Calories per serving: ~195 (without whipped cream; varies with milk/yogurt choice).

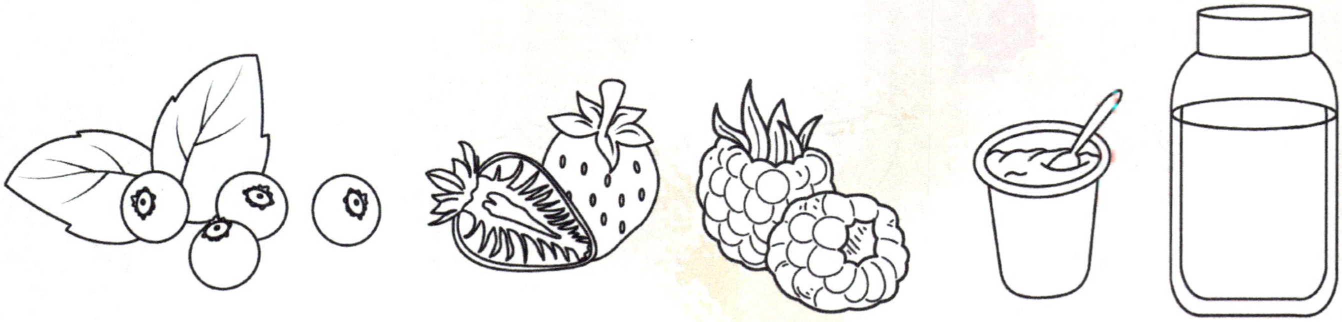

Your body now follows a rhythm: solid fuel in the morning, light nourishment at night. It's the perfect balance for digestion, weight, and peace of mind. Lightness feels natural now.

Tropical Mango Banana Smoothie Ingredients (Serves 2):

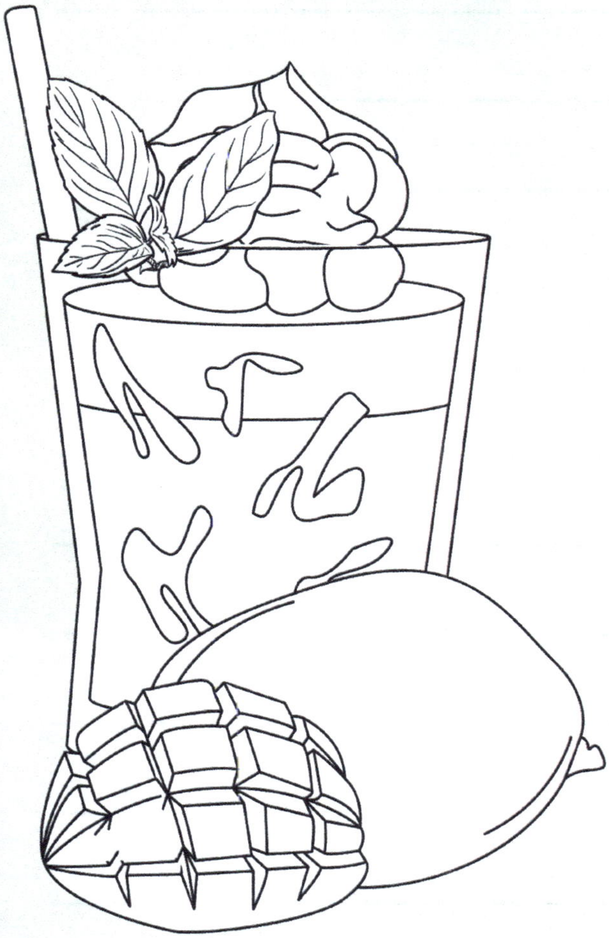

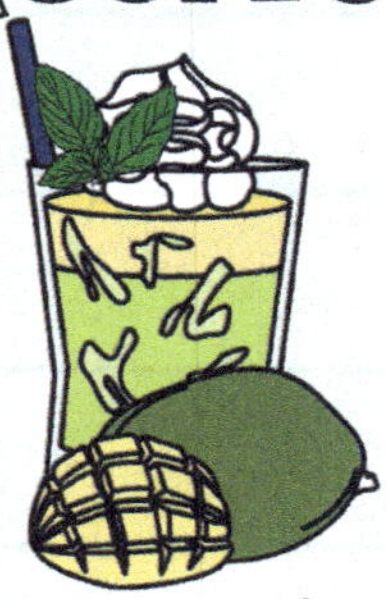

- 1 cup frozen mango chunks: Bursting with vitamins A + C for immune support.
- 1 ripe banana: Natural sweetness + potassium for muscle function.
- ½ cup Greek yogurt: Probiotics + protein (use coconut yogurt for vegan).
- ½ cup orange juice: Freshly squeezed for vitamin C + tangy brightness.

Whipped cream (optional): For a decadent finishing touch.
Ice cubes: For a frosty, refreshing texture.

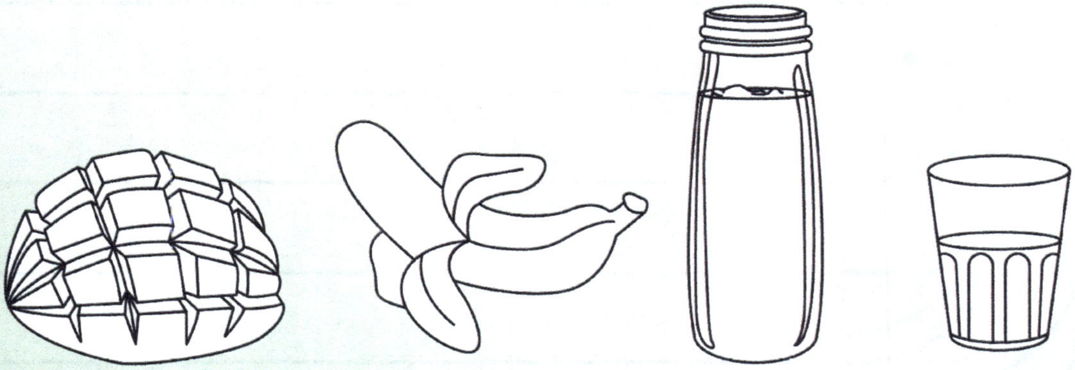

My Notes & Ideas

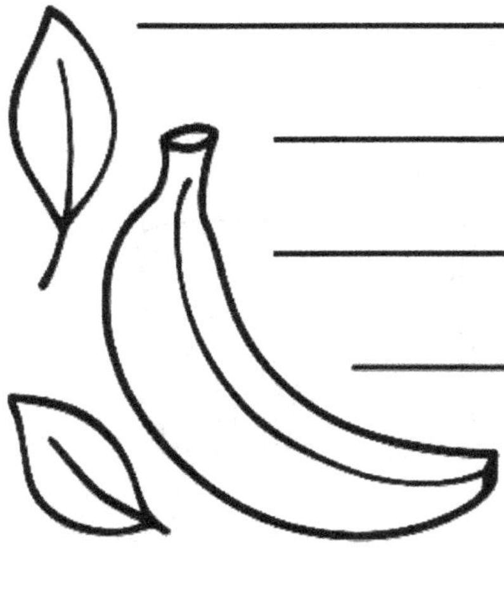

Weekly Wellness Check-In

Weight This Week ______________________

____

____

Favorite Smoothie ________________

____

____

Mood This Week ______________________

____

____

Notes ________________________

____

Day 22 - New Balance

Smoothies for breakfast and dinner, high-protein lunch.

Green Detox Smoothie Ingredients (Serves 2):

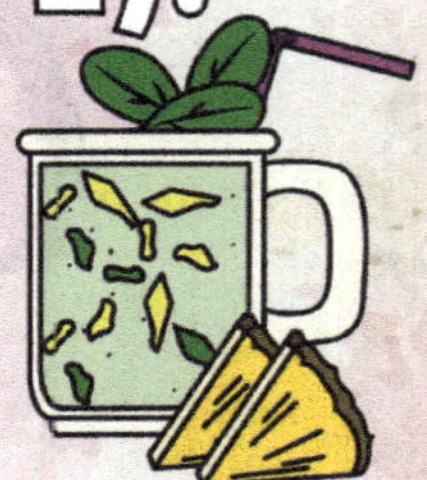

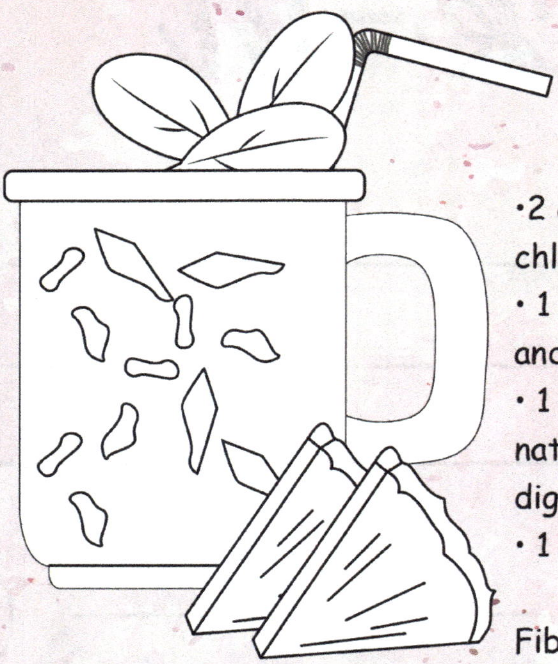

•2 cups fresh spinach: Rich in iron, chlorophyll, and vitamins A/C.
• 1 cup cucumber (chopped): Hydrating and loaded with silica for skin health.
• 1 cup frozen pineapple chunks: Adds natural sweetness + bromelain for digestion.
• 1 cup apple (cored and chopped):

Fiber-rich with quercetin for immunity.
Juice of 1 lemon (~2 tbsp): Detoxifying and high in vitamin C.
1 cup coconut water: Replenishes electrolytes naturally.

Ice cubes: For a frosty, thirst-quenching texture.
250 calories

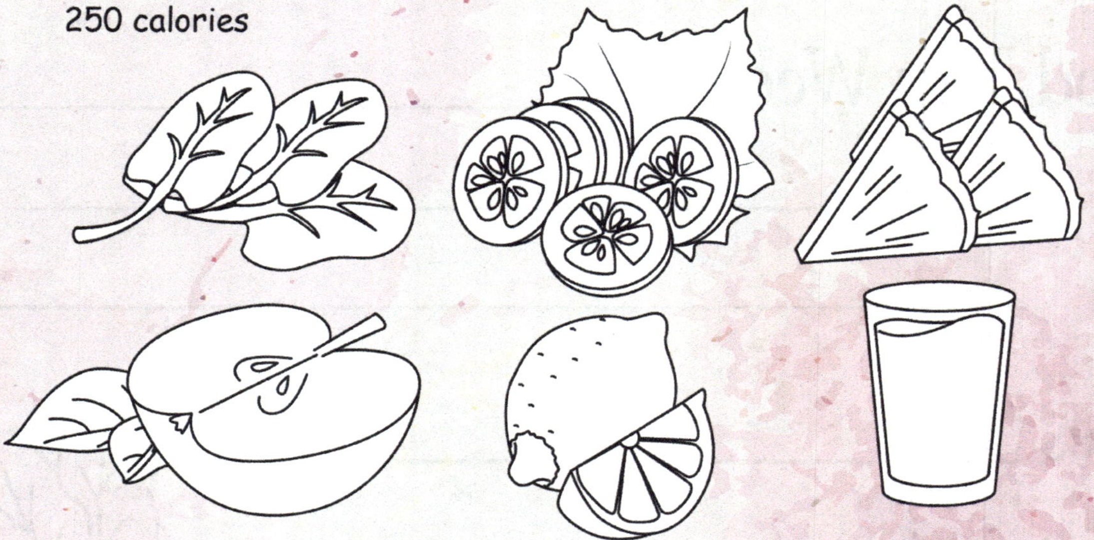

Your body adjusts to light meals in the morning and evening, while lunch provides the protein needed for energy and recovery.

Raspberry Coconut Smoothie Ingredients (Serves 2):

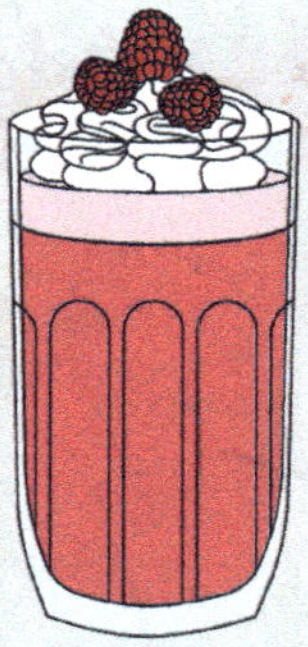

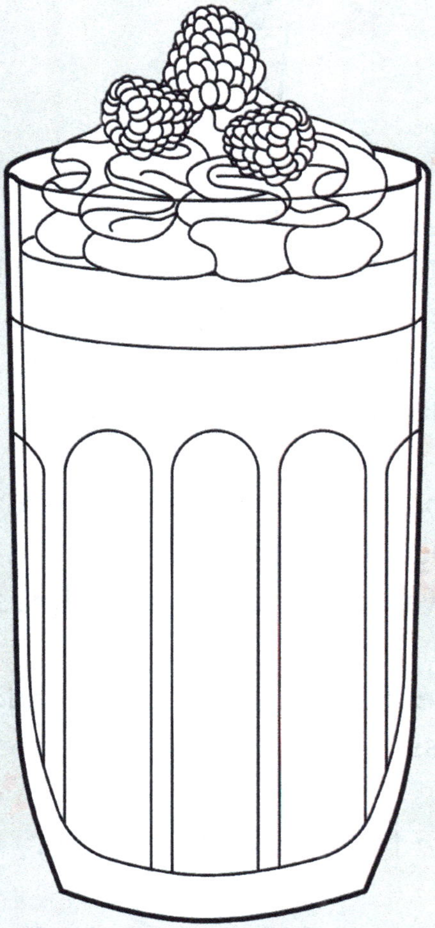

- 1 cup frozen raspberries: High in antioxidants and fiber.
- $\frac{1}{2}$ cup coconut milk: Full-fat for creaminess or light for fewer calories.
- $\frac{1}{2}$ cup Greek yogurt: Probiotics + protein (use coconut yogurt for vegan).
- Ice cubes: For a frosty, hydrating texture.

Calories per serving: ~240 (varies with yogurt and juice choices).

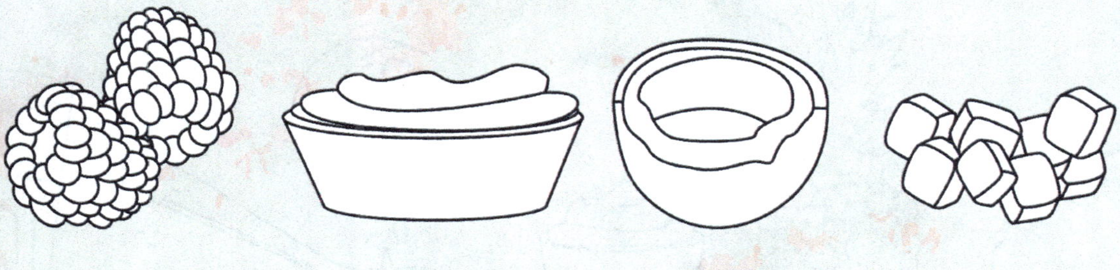

Day 23 - Stable Energy

Smoothies for breakfast and dinner, high-protein lunch.

Mango Pineapple Smoothie

Ingredients (Serves 2):

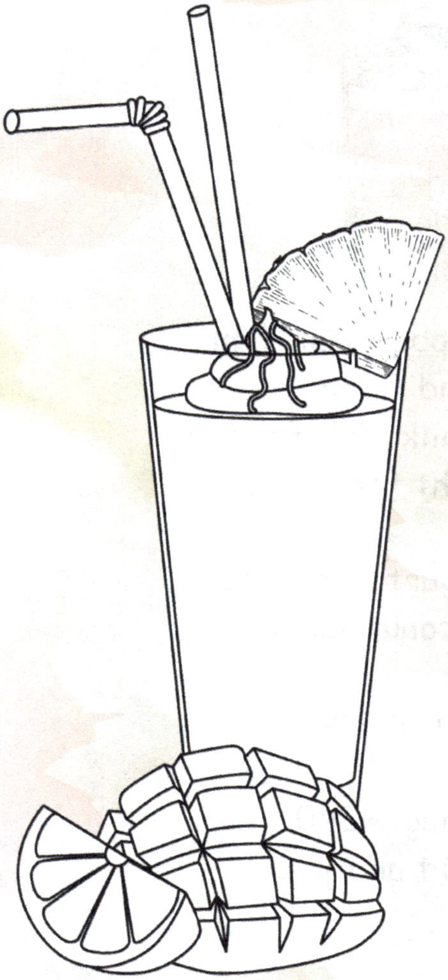

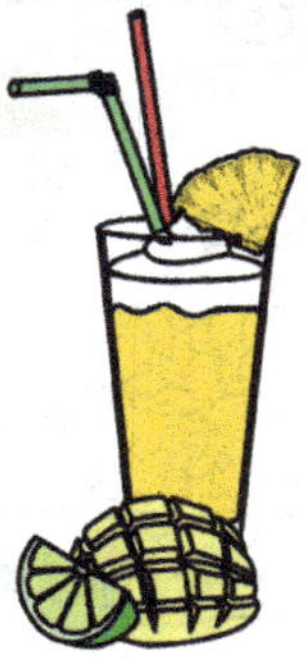

• 1 cup frozen mango chunks: High in vitamin C + beta-carotene for glowing skin.

•1 cup frozen pineapple chunks: Contains bromelain to ease digestion + reduce bloating.

•$\frac{1}{2}$ cup Greek yogurt: Probiotics + 12g protein (use coconut yogurt for vegan).

$\frac{1}{2}$ cup coconut water: Natural electrolytes for hydration.

1 tbsp lime juice: Enhances immunity + adds zesty brightness.

Ice cubes: For a frosty, slushy texture.

Calories per serving: ~140 (varies with yogurt and coconut water choices).

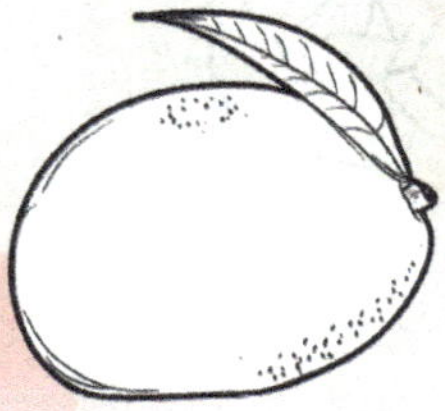
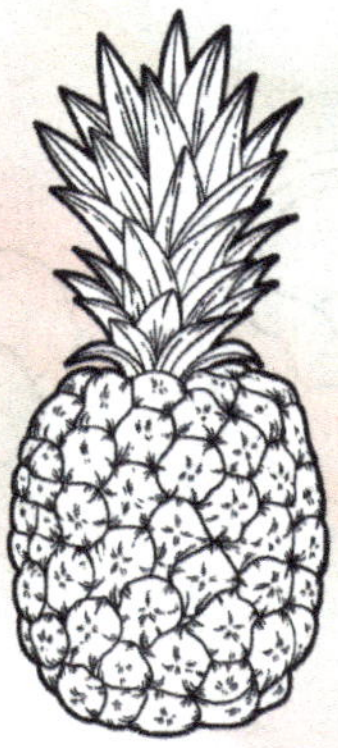
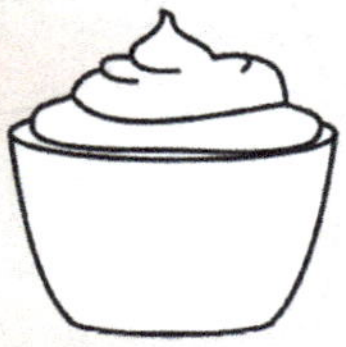
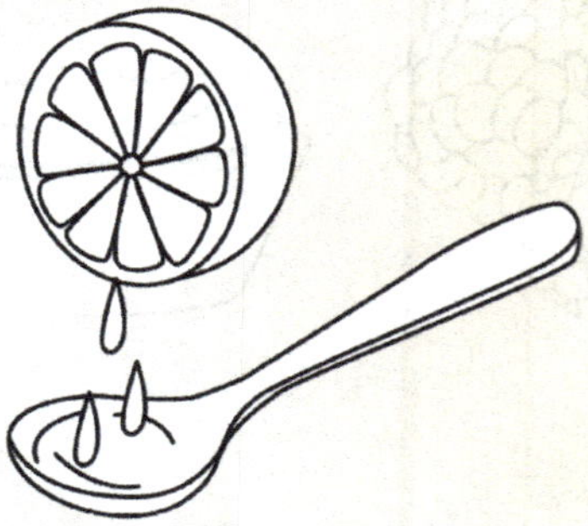
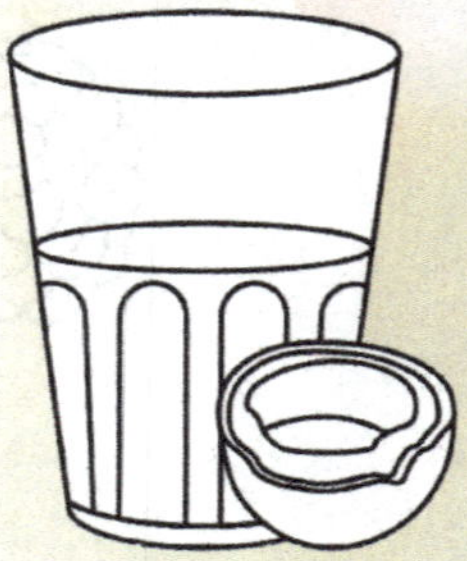

Protein supports muscle maintenance and curbs hunger. Smoothies digest easily, giving you comfort and lightness.

Blueberry Spinach Smoothie Ingredients (Serves 2):

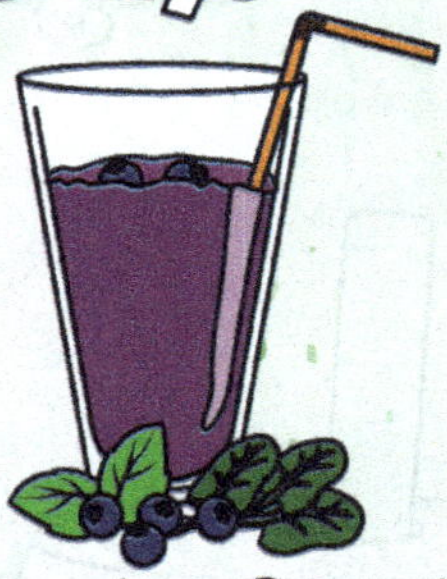

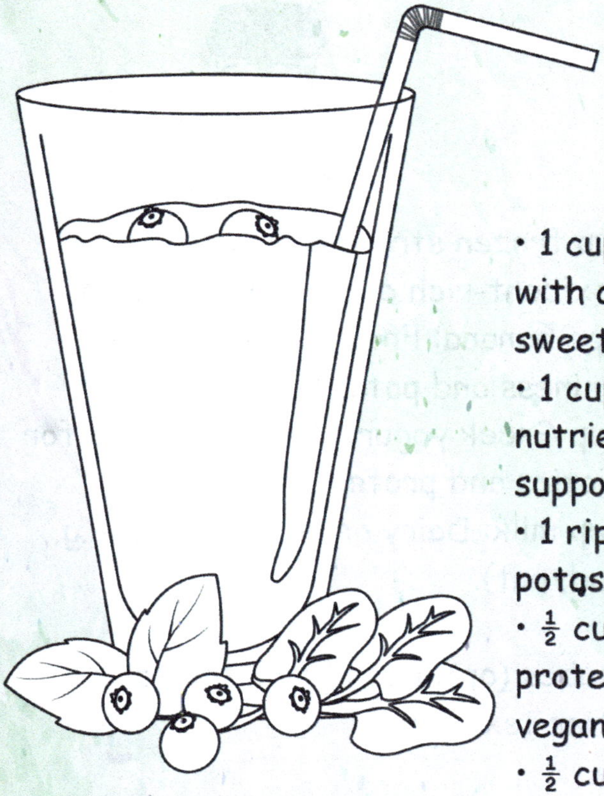

- 1 cup frozen blueberries: Bursting with antioxidants and natural sweetness.
- 1 cup fresh spinach: Mild, nutrient-dense greens for detox support.
- 1 ripe banana: Adds creaminess and potassium.
- ½ cup Greek yogurt: Probiotics + protein (use plant-based yogurt for vegan).
- ½ cup milk: Dairy or plant-based (e.g., almond, oat).

Ice cubes (optional): For a frostier texture.

Calories: ~150

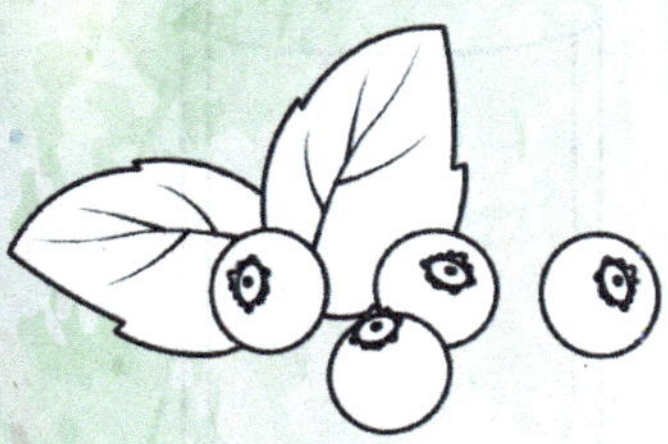
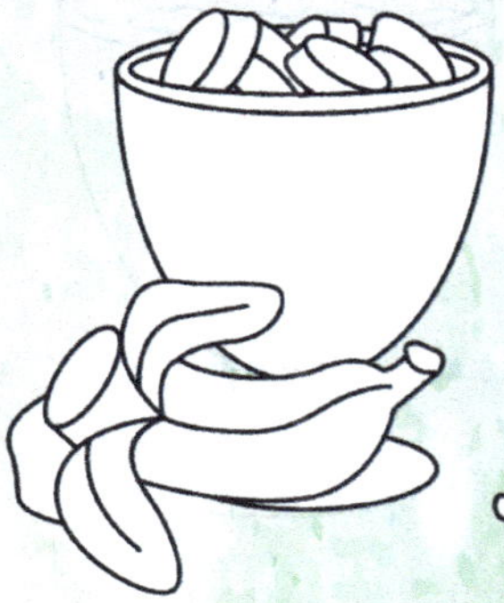
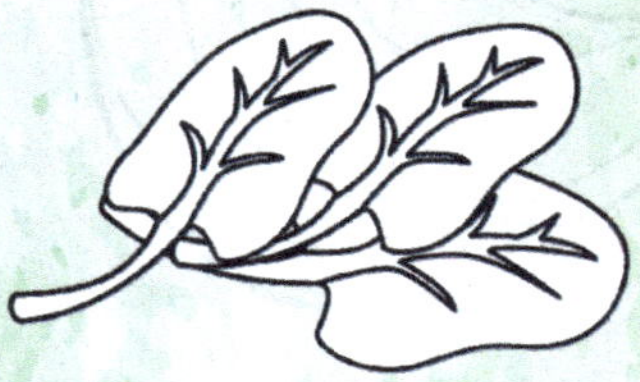
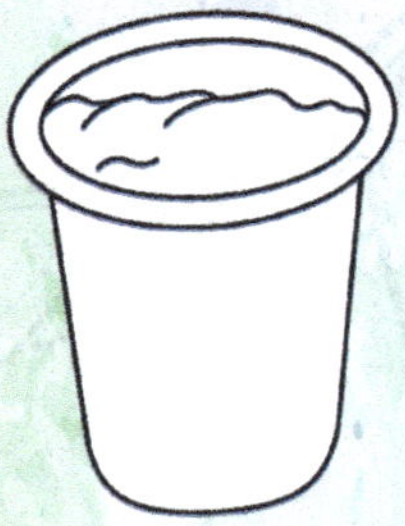
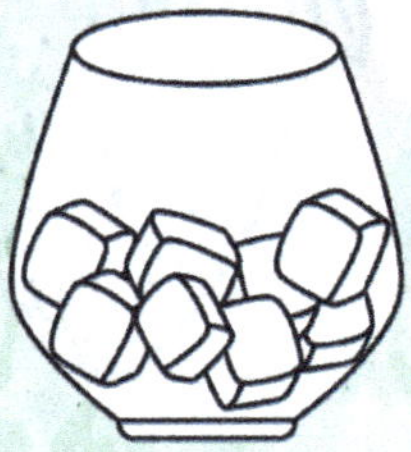

Day 24 - Improved Digestion

Smoothies for breakfast and dinner, high-protein lunch.

Strawberry Banana Smoothie
Ingredients (Serves 2):

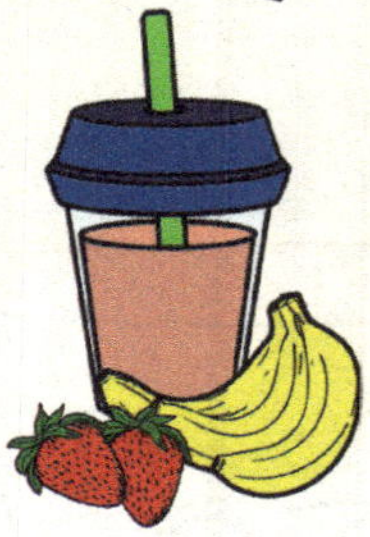

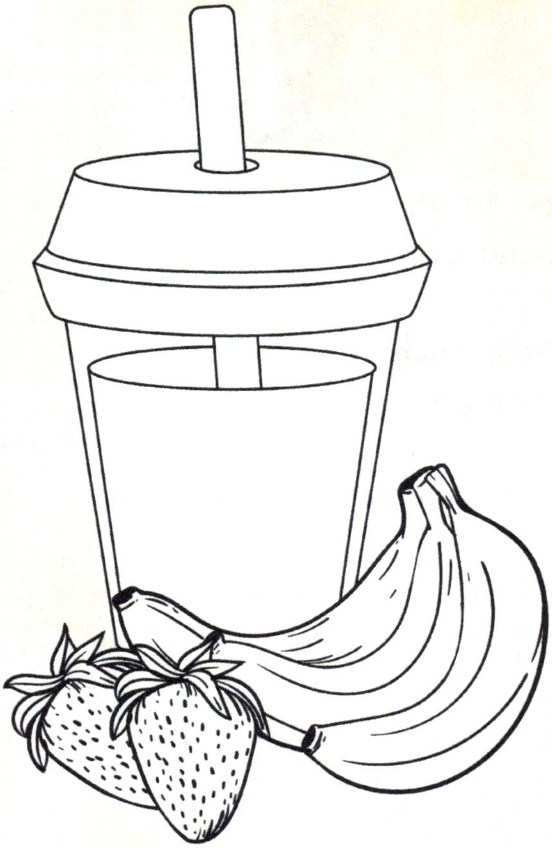

- 1 cup frozen strawberries: Antioxidant-rich and naturally sweet.
- 1 ripe banana: Fresh or frozen for creaminess and potassium.
- $\frac{1}{2}$ cup Greek yogurt: Plain or vanilla for probiotics and protein.
- $\frac{1}{2}$ cup milk: Dairy or plant-based (e.g., almond, oat).

Ice cubes (optional): For a thicker, frostier texture.

Calories: ~95

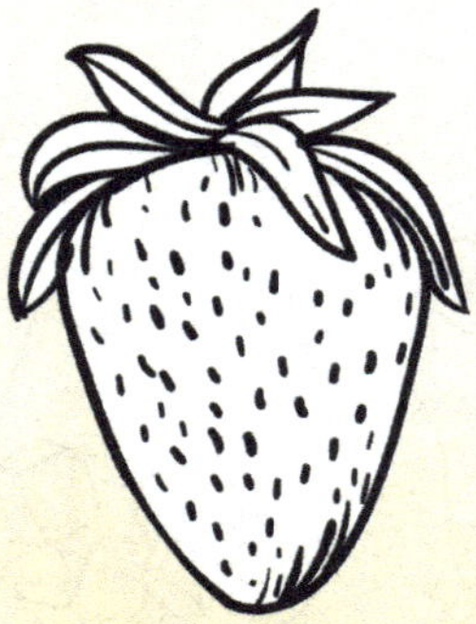

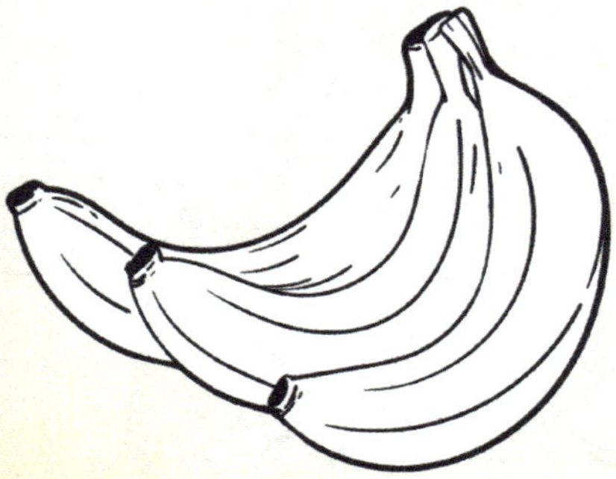

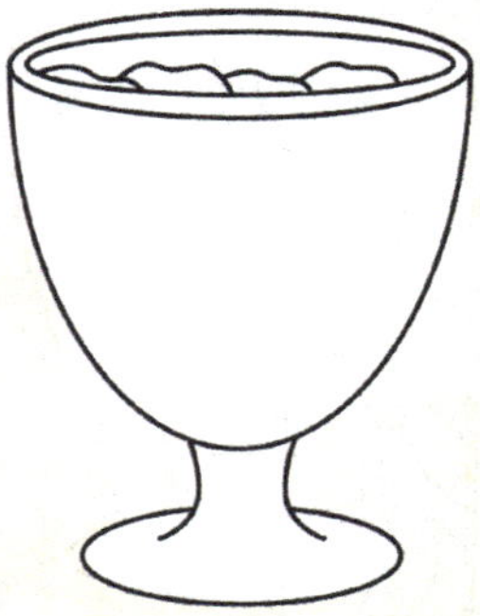

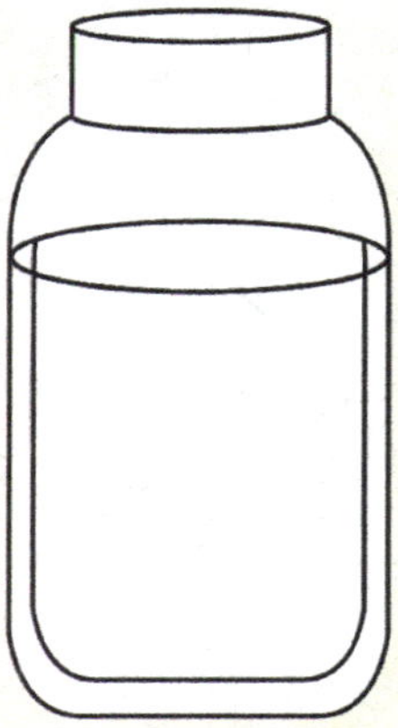

This routine helps prevent overeating. Your digestive system works smoothly without heaviness or discomfort.

Mango Spinach Smoothie:

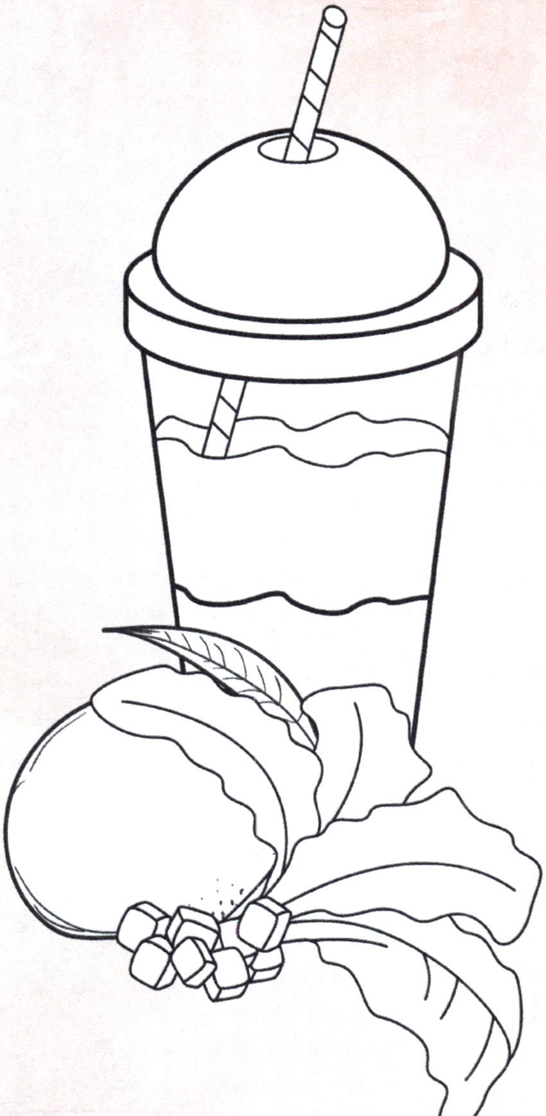

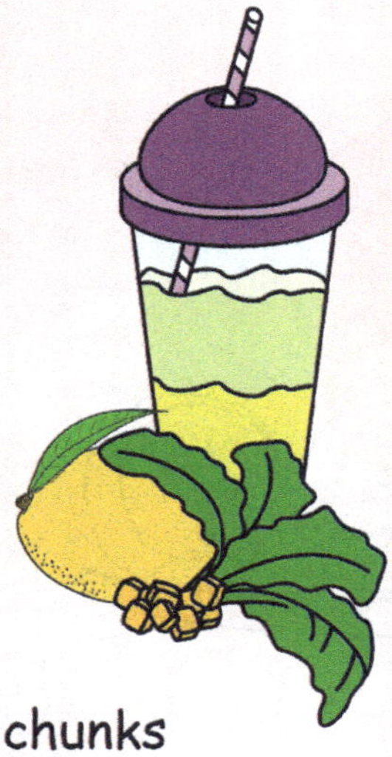

- 1 cup mango chunks
- 2 cups baby spinach
- 1 cup unsweetened almond milk
- 1 frozen banana
- 1 tsp honey (optional)

Calories: ~135 per serving

Benefits: Combines vitamin C-rich mango and iron-packed spinach for immunity and energy.

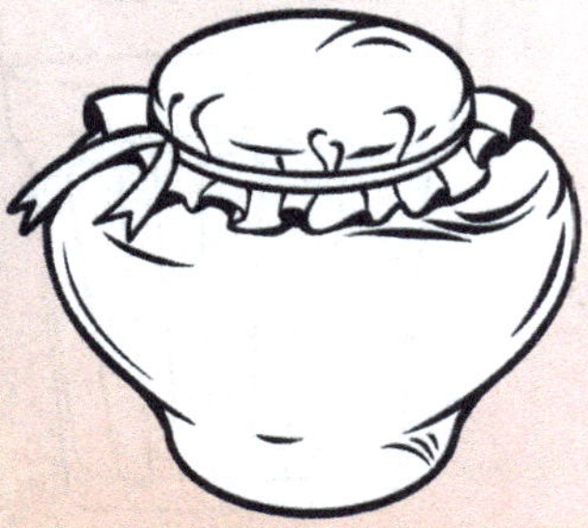

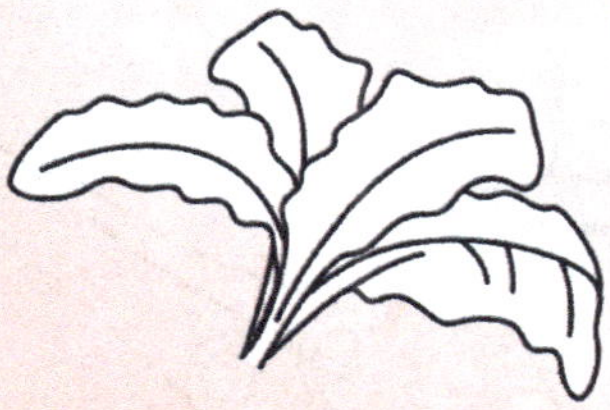

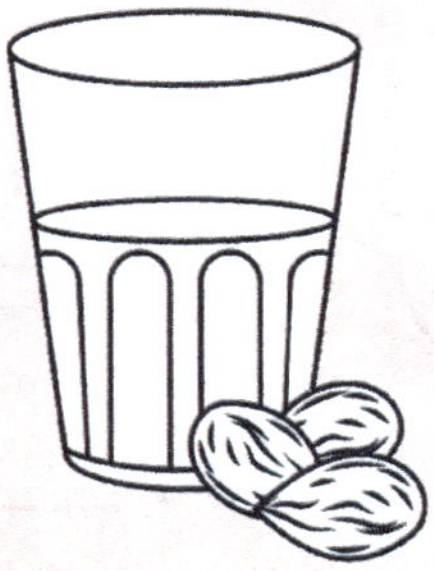

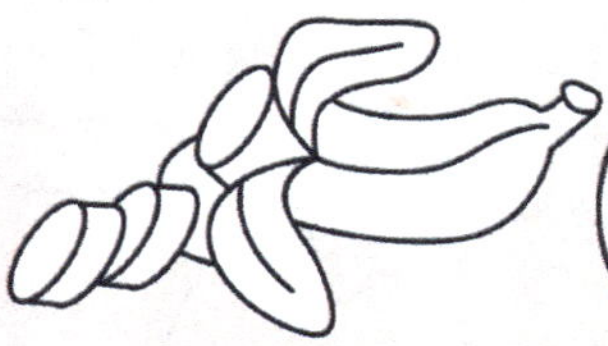

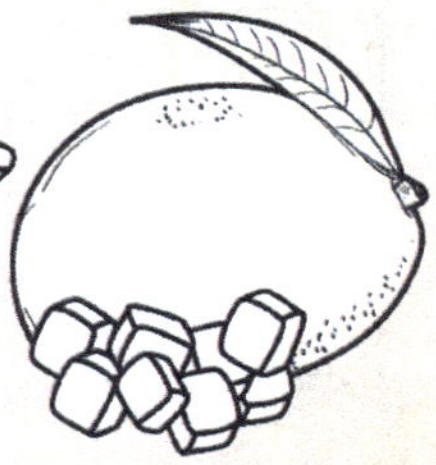

Day 25 – Muscle Support and Recovery
Smoothies for breakfast and dinner, high-protein lunch.

Peanut Butter Banana Smoothie:

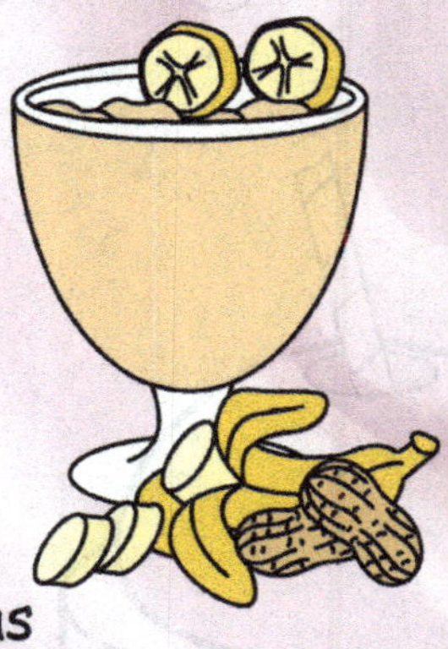

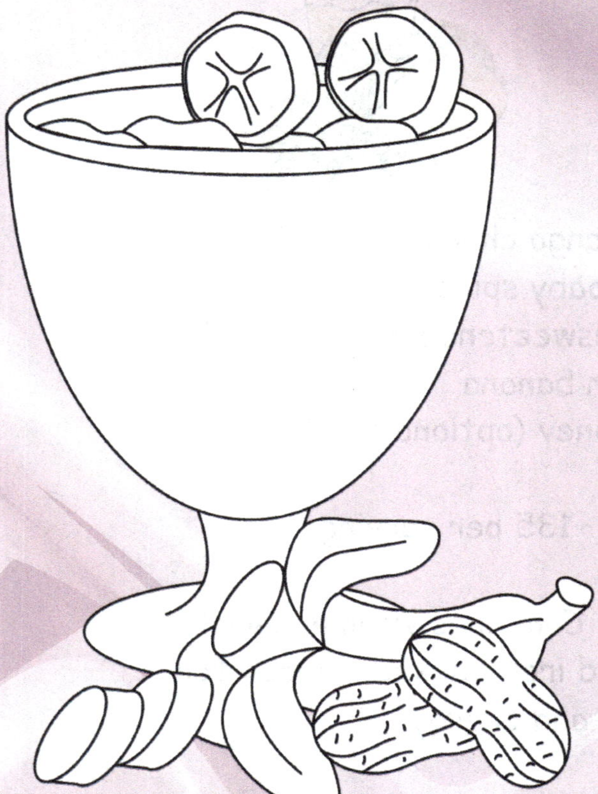

- 2 ripe bananas
- 2 tbsp natural peanut butter
- ½ cup Greek yogurt
- 1 cup milk (dairy or plant-based)
- ½ tsp cinnamon

Calories: ~250 per serving

Benefits: Protein-packed with peanut butter and Greek yogurt to repair muscles and curb hunger.

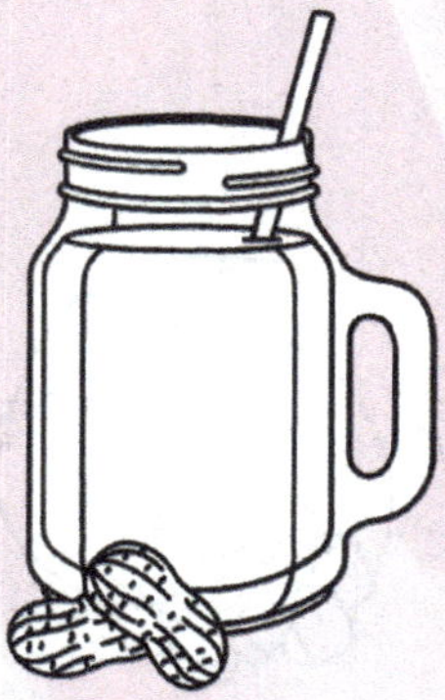

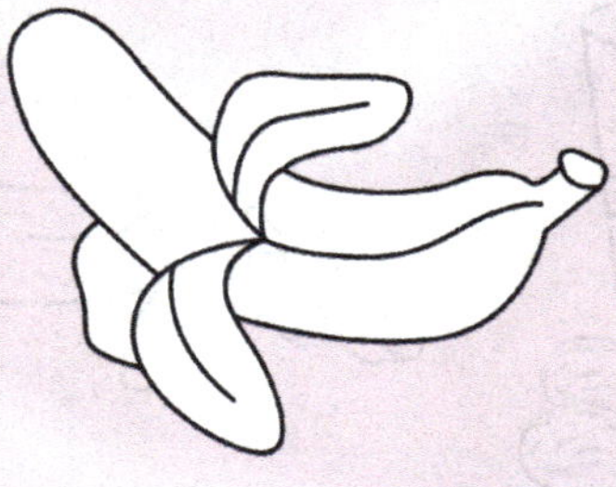

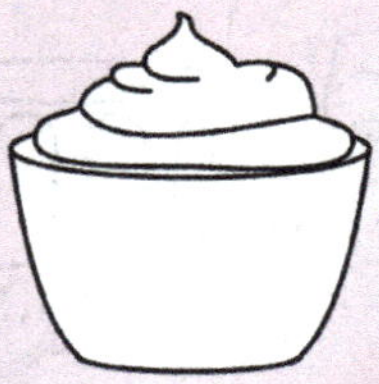

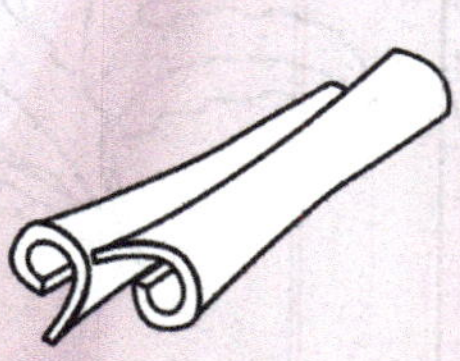

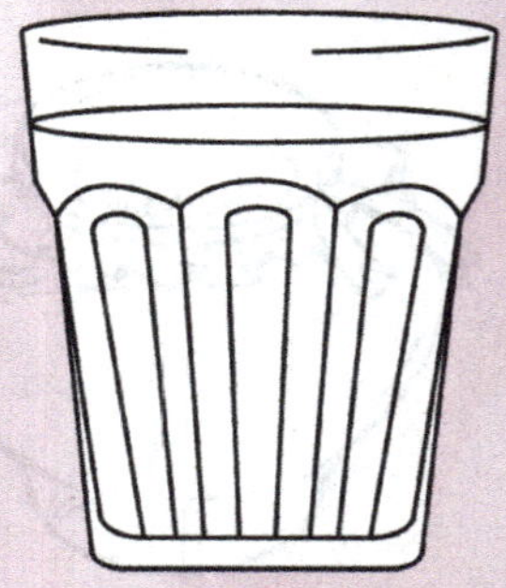

Smoothie Queen

High-protein lunch supports muscle growth and repair. Smoothies keep your stomach light and free from overload.

Chocolate Berry Smoothie:

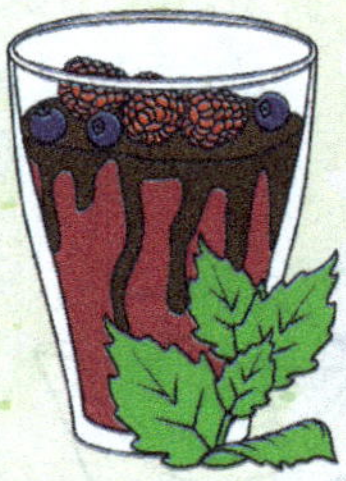

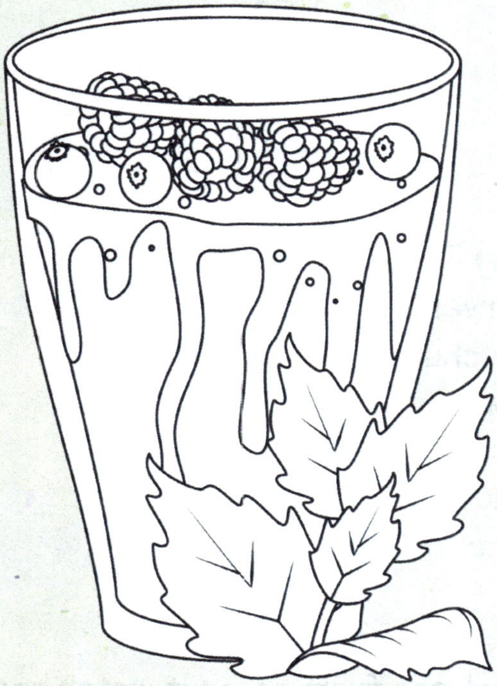

Mood: Guilt-Free Dessert Craving

Ingredients (Serves 2):

- 1 cup frozen mixed berries
- 1-2 tbsp unsweetened cocoa powder
- 1 cup almond milk
- $\frac{1}{2}$ cup Greek yogurt
- 1-2 tsp honey

Calories: ~105 per serving

Benefits: Antioxidant-rich berries and heart-healthy cocoa satisfy sweet cravings.

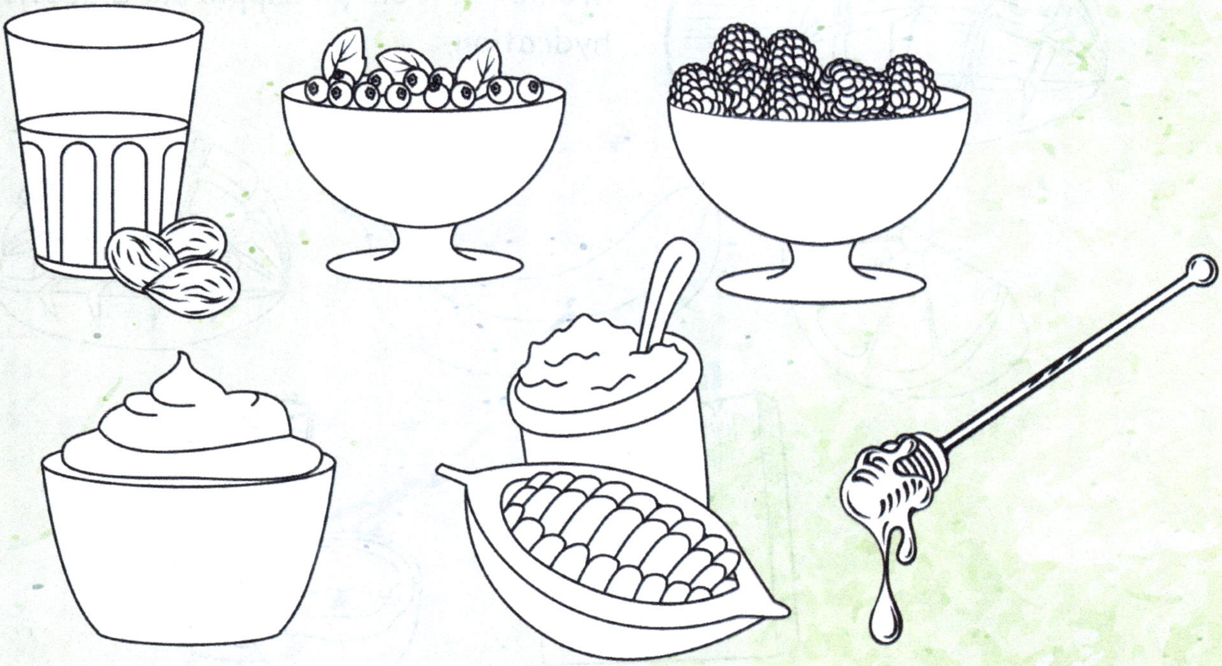

Day 26 – Reduced Inflammation

Smoothies for breakfast and dinner, high-protein lunch.

Tropical Delight Smoothie:

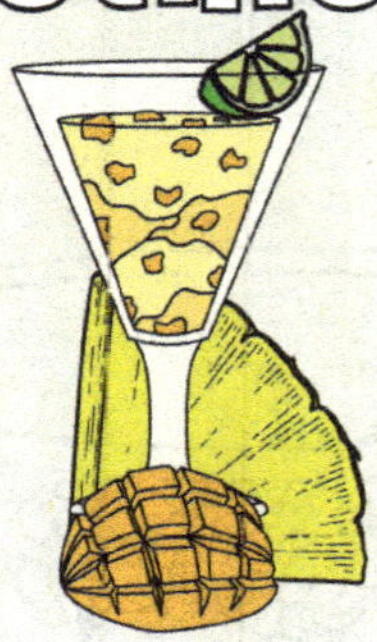

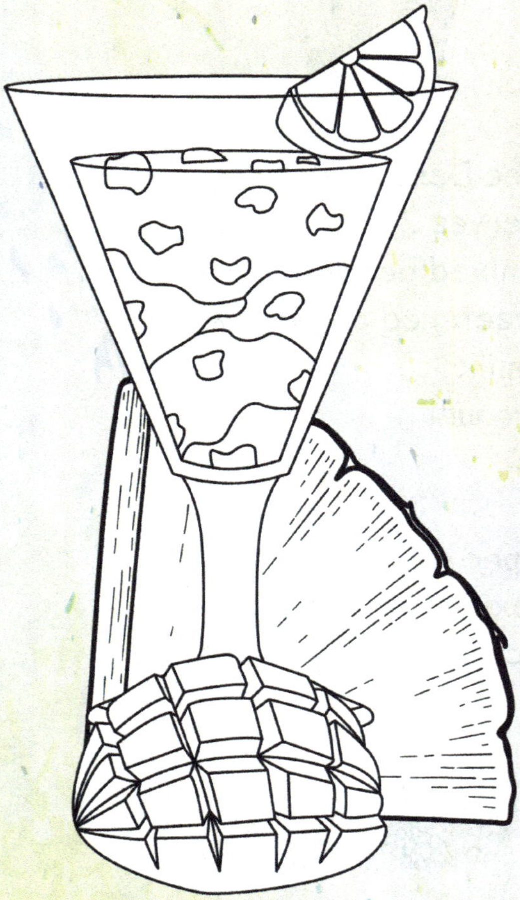

Mood: Hydrating Tropical Escape

Ingredients (Serves 2):

- 1 cup pineapple chunks
- 1 cup coconut water
- 1 cup mango
- 1 frozen banana
- 1 tbsp lime juice

Calories: ~170 per serving

Benefits: Electrolytes from coconut water and bromelain from pineapple aid digestion and hydration.

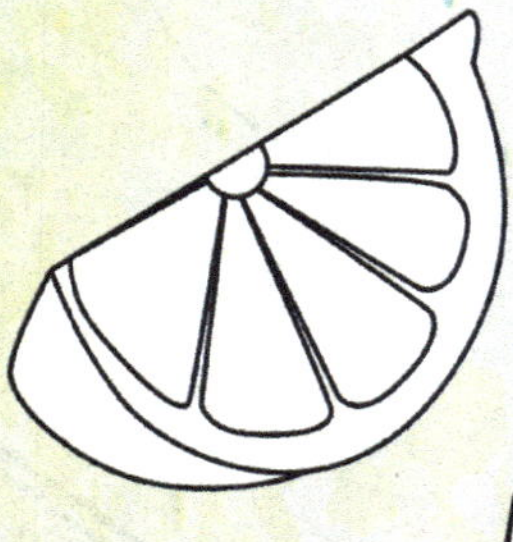

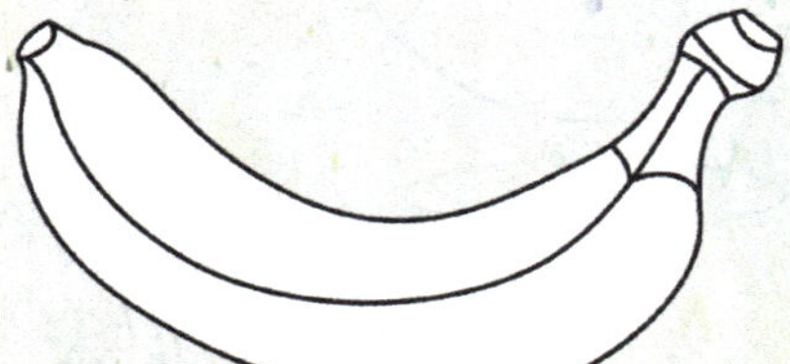

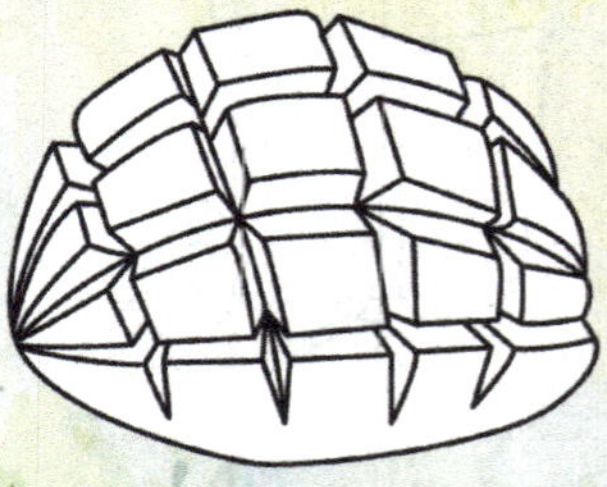

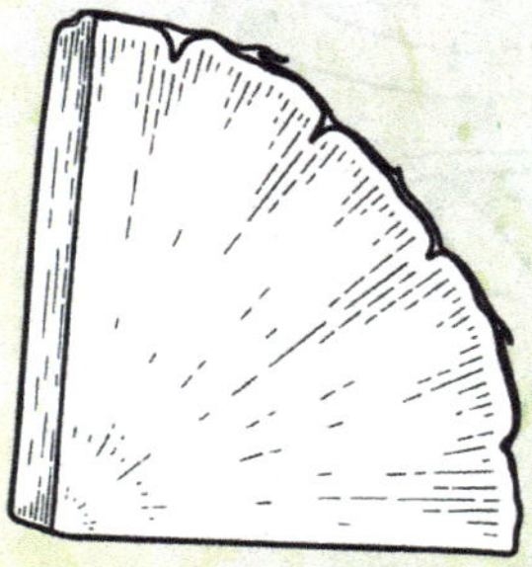

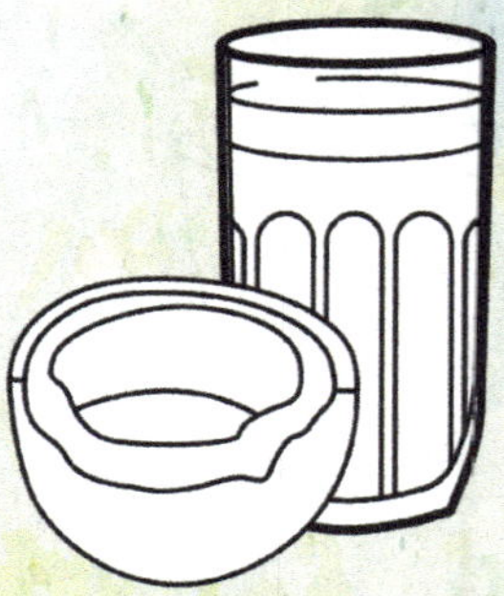

This plan helps lower internal inflammation, improving overall wellbeing and tone.

Avocado Green Goodness Smoothie:

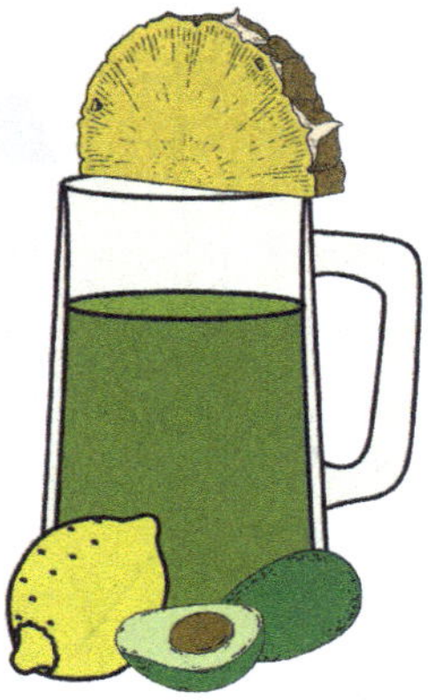

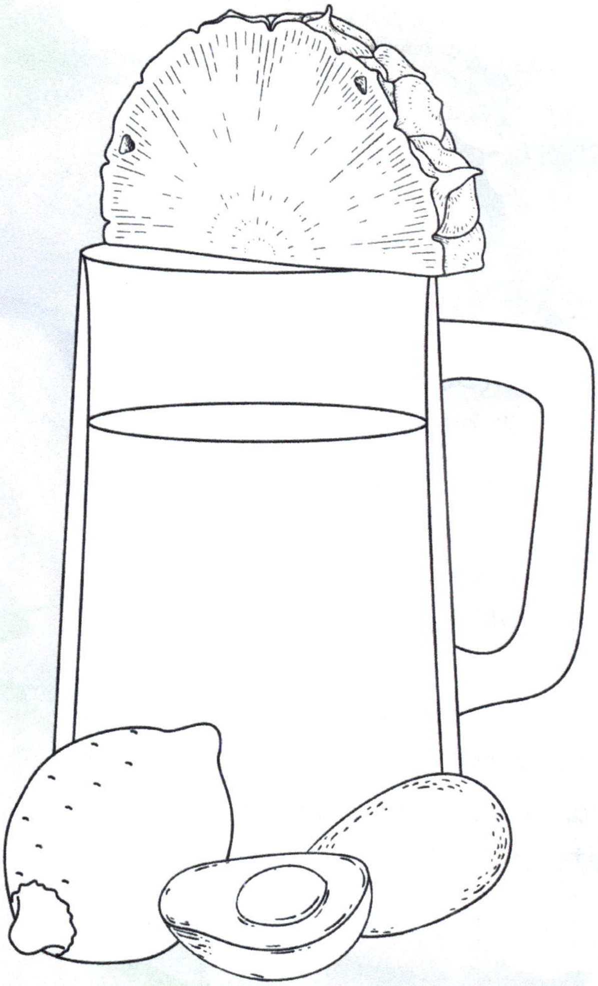

Mood: Creamy Detox & Glow

Ingredients (Serves 2):

- 1 ripe avocado
- 2 cups baby spinach
- 1 cup frozen pineapple
- 1 cup coconut milk
- 1 tbsp lemon juice

Calories: ~390 per serving (with full-fat coconut milk)

Benefits: Healthy fats from avocado and detoxifying spinach nourish skin and liver.

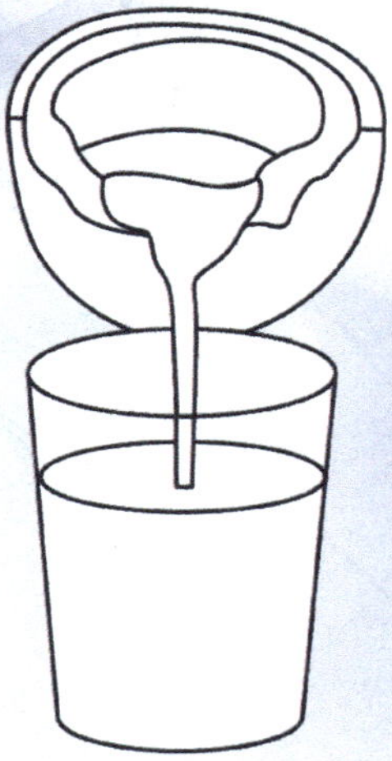

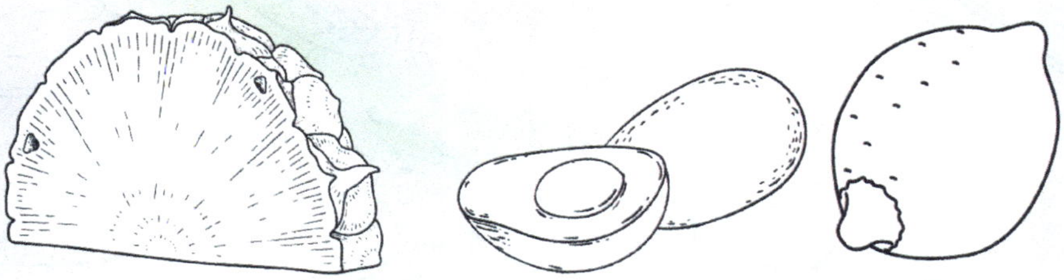

Day 27 - Feeling Light and Strong

Smoothies for breakfast and dinner, high-protein lunch.

Carrot Orange Smoothie:

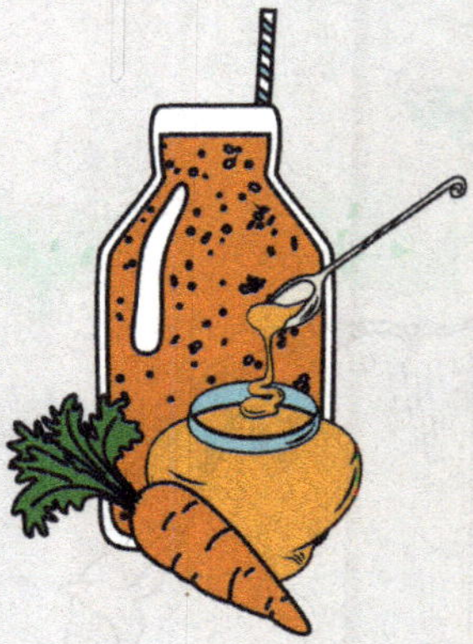

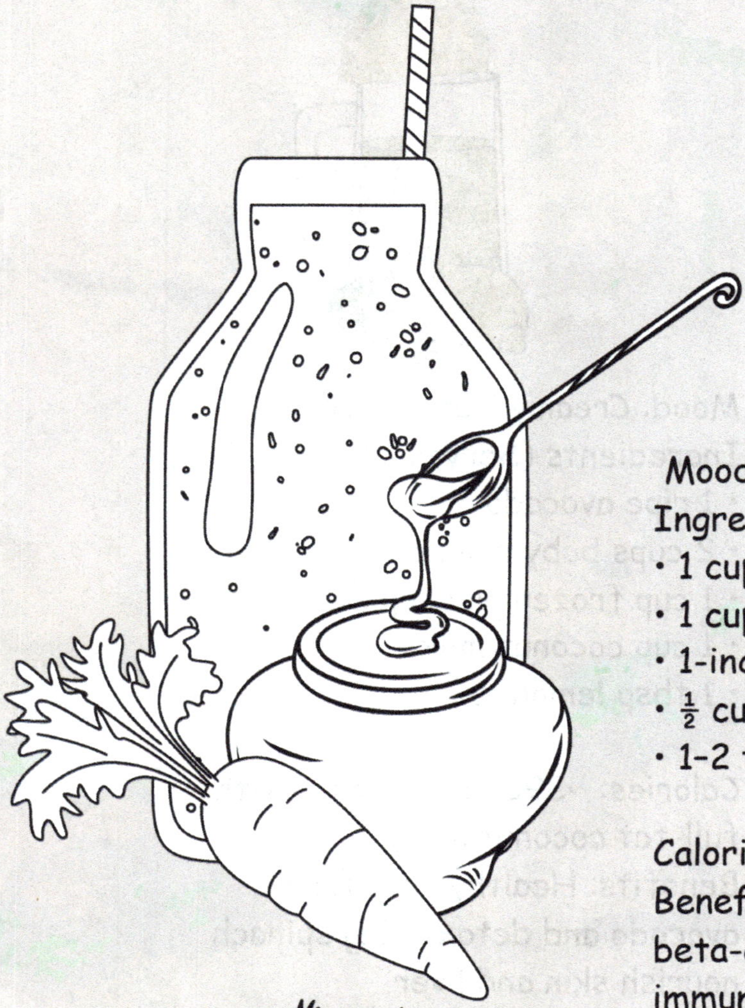

Mood: Immunity-Boosting Zest

Ingredients (Serves 2):

- 1 cup fresh orange juice
- 1 cup shredded carrots
- 1-inch fresh ginger
- ½ cup Greek yogurt
- 1-2 tsp honey

Calories: ~130 per serving

Benefits: Vitamin C from oranges and beta-carotene from carrots support immunity and vision.

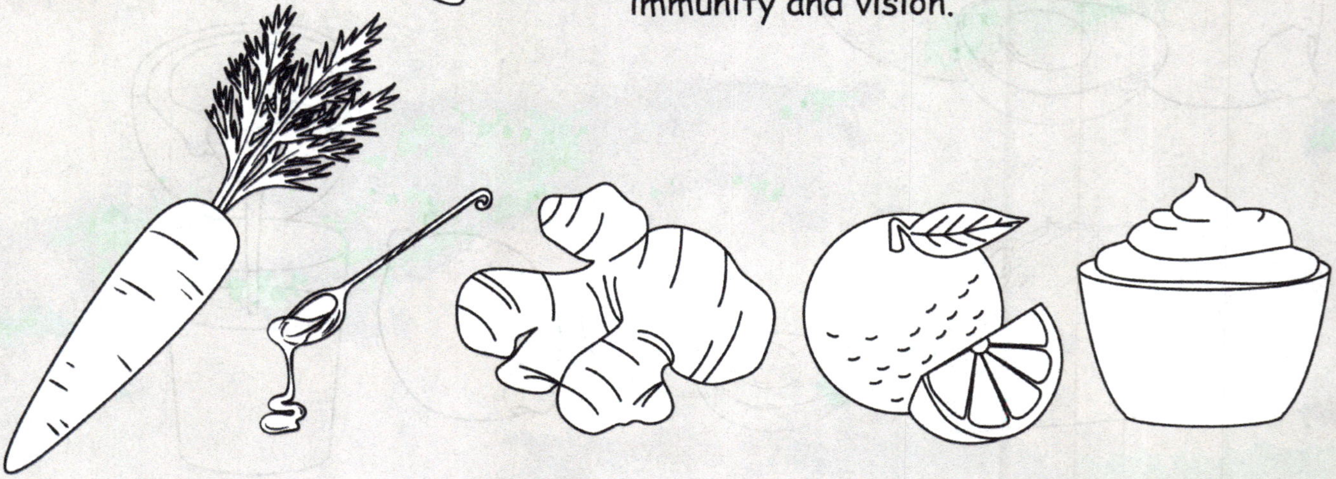

You feel energized, light in your body, and emotionally balanced.

Super Energy Charger Recipe:

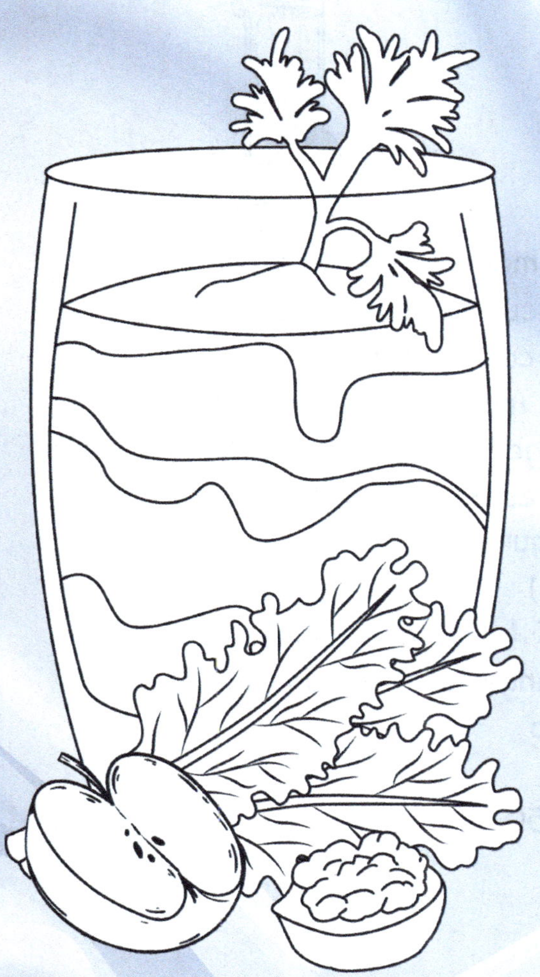

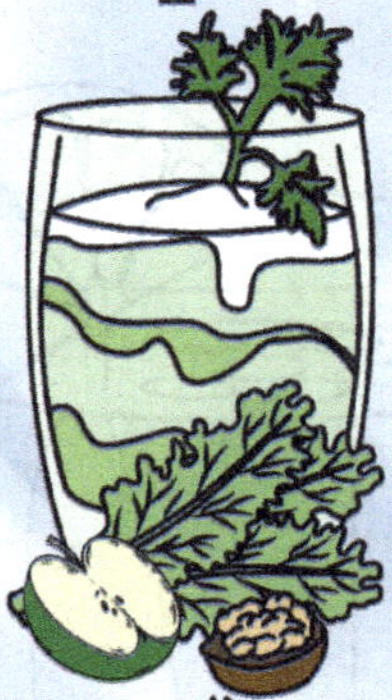

- Kale: 2 cups (ribs removed) (chlorophyll)
- Banana: ½ medium (slow-release carbs)
- Green apple: ½ cup (quercetin)
- Avocado: ½ (healthy fats)
- Pineapple: ½ cup (manganese)
- Parsley: 1 handful (vitamin K)
- Walnuts: 1 tbsp (omega-3s)
- Coconut water: 1¼ cup (electrolytes)
- Lemon juice: 1 tbsp (vitamin C)
- Ice: ½ cup

Calories: ~420

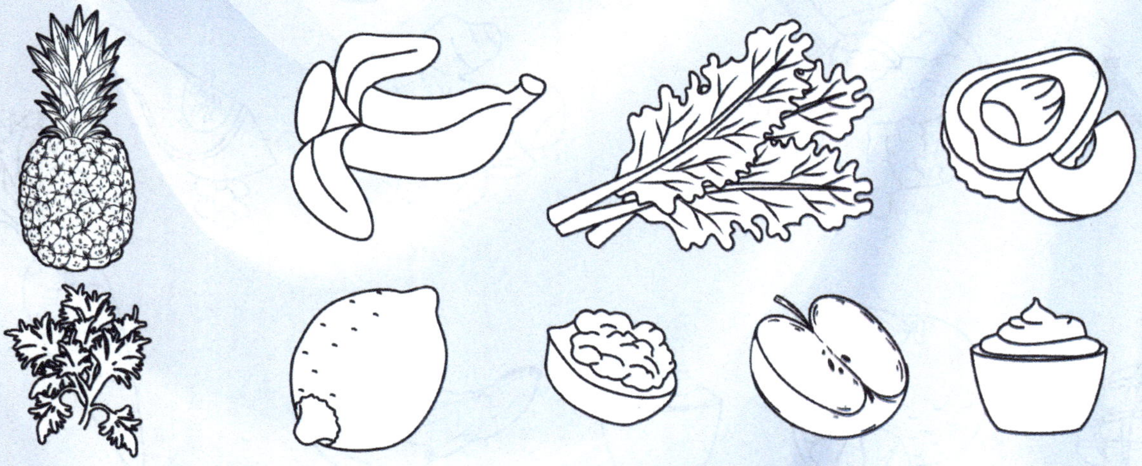

Day 28 – Optimal Balance

Smoothies for breakfast and dinner, high-protein lunch.

Anti-Inflammatory Smoothie Recipe:

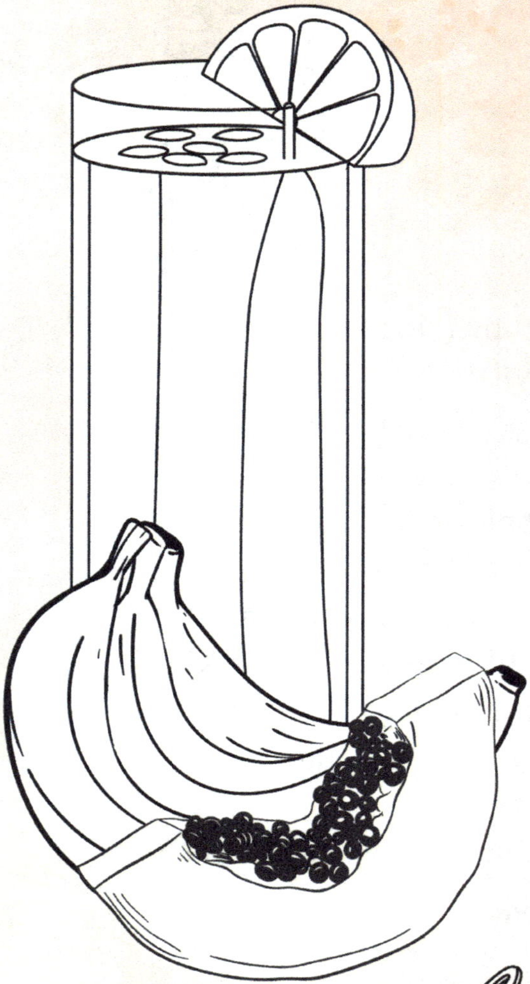

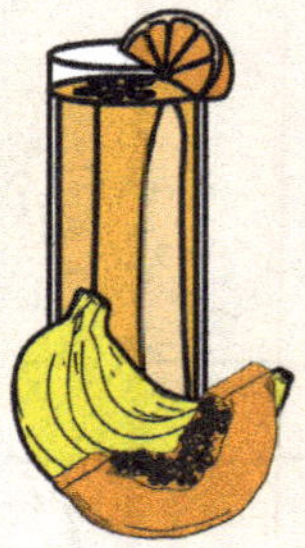

- Carrot: 1 medium (beta-carotene)
- Papaya: 1 cup (digestive enzymes)
- Mango: $\frac{1}{2}$ cup (vitamin C)
- Banana: $\frac{1}{2}$ medium (potassium)
- Fresh ginger: 1" piece (gingerols)
- Pumpkin seeds: 1 tbsp (zinc)
- Greek yogurt: 1 scoop ($\frac{1}{4}$ cup) (probiotics)
- Turmeric: $\frac{1}{2}$ tsp (curcumin)
- Fresh orange juice: $\frac{3}{4}$ cup (liquid base)
- Ice: $\frac{1}{2}$ cup

Calories: 350

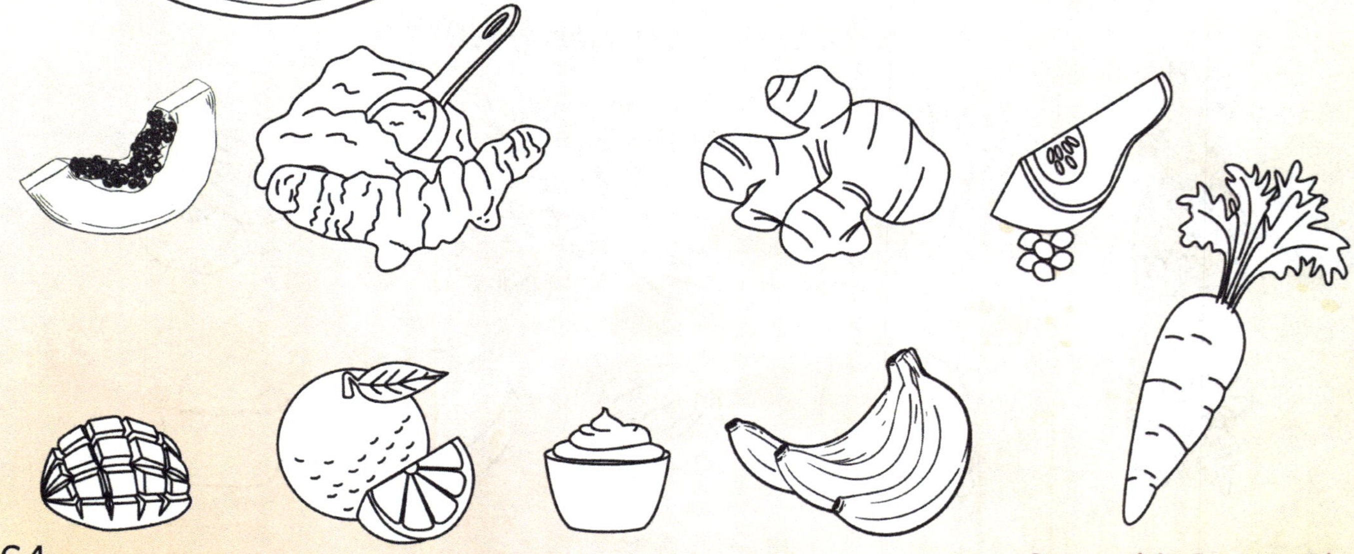

Your body is fully adapted to this rhythm. Energy and digestion are at their best, and your body feels harmonious and strong.

Vitamin C Monster Recipe:

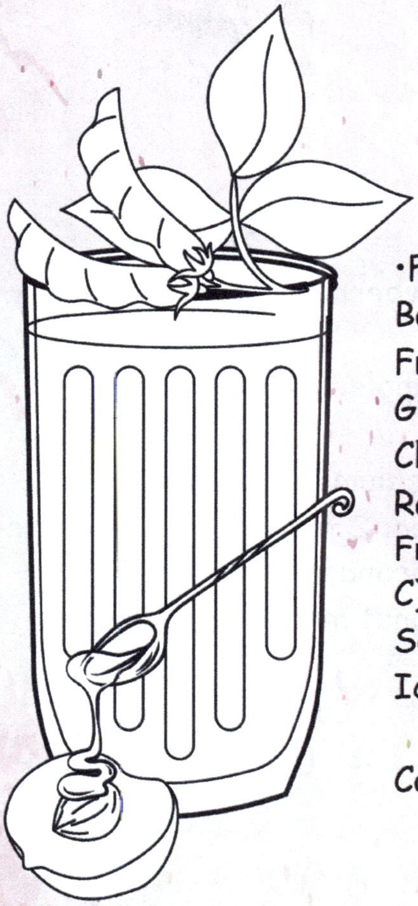

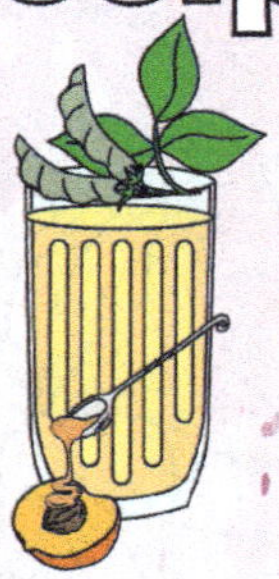

•Frozen mango: $\frac{1}{2}$ cup (101% DV vitamin C)
Banana: $\frac{1}{2}$ medium (potassium)
Frozen peaches: $\frac{1}{2}$ cup (17% DV vitamin C)
Greek yogurt: 1 scoop ($\frac{1}{4}$ cup) (probiotics)
Chia seeds: 1 tbsp (omega-3s)
Raw honey: 1 tbsp (enzymes)
Fresh orange juice: $\frac{1}{4}$ cup (62% DV vitamin C)
Soy milk: $\frac{1}{4}$ cup (plant protein)
Ice: $\frac{1}{2}$ cup

Calories: 380

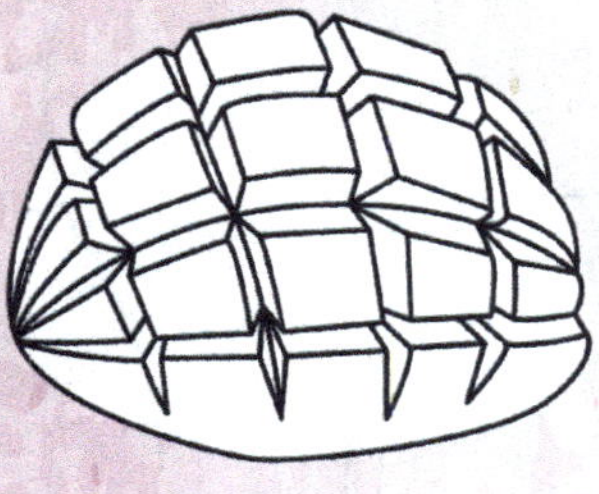

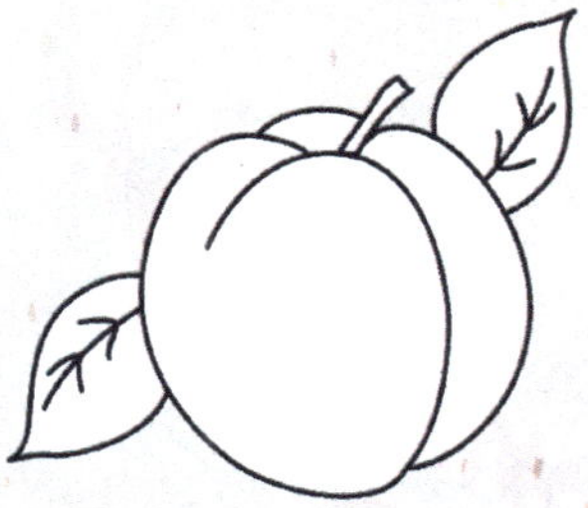

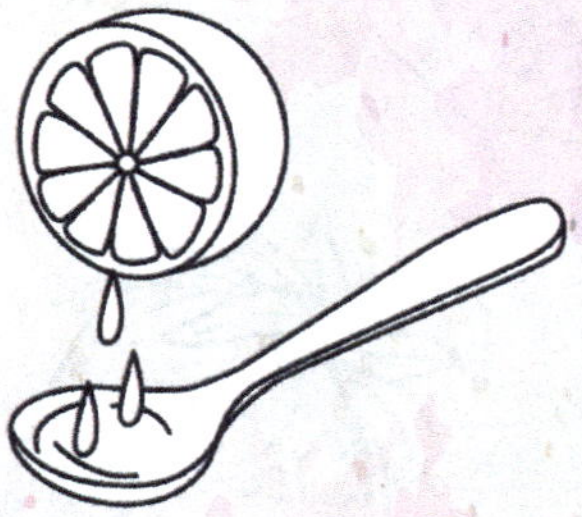

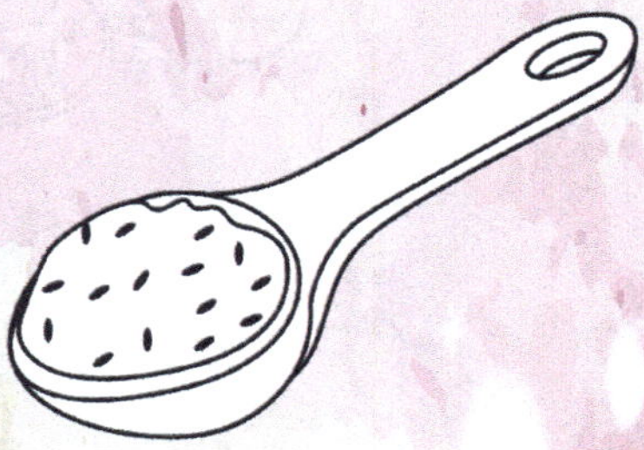

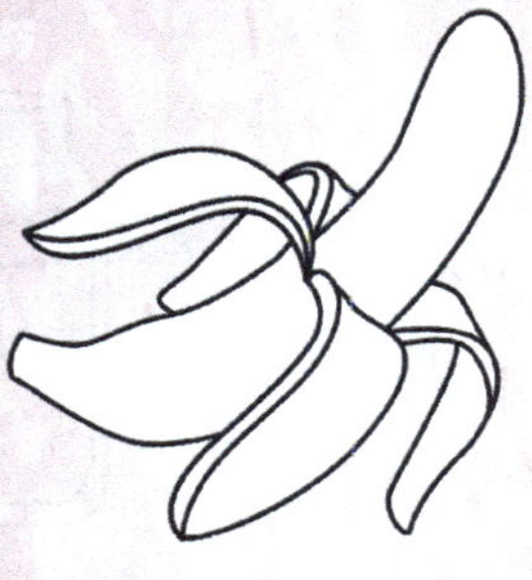

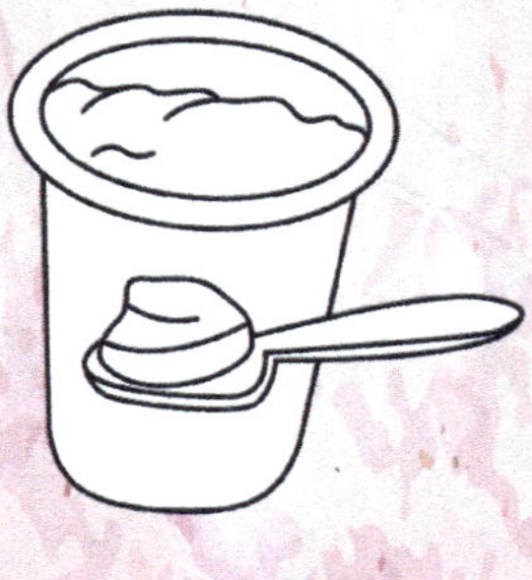

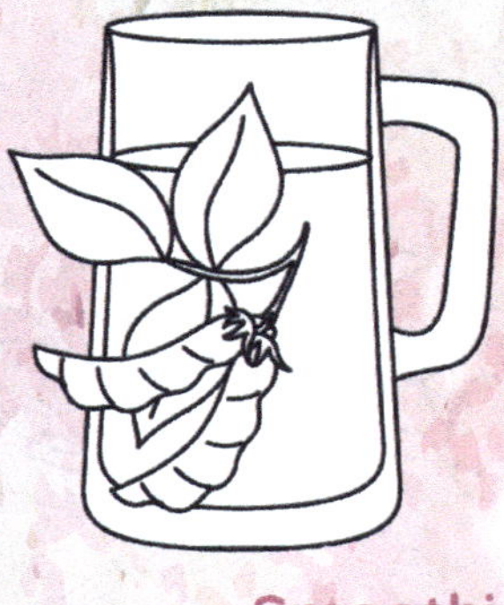

Day 29 - Inner Harmony

Smoothies for breakfast and dinner, high-protein lunch.

Pink Aloha Protein Power Smoothie:

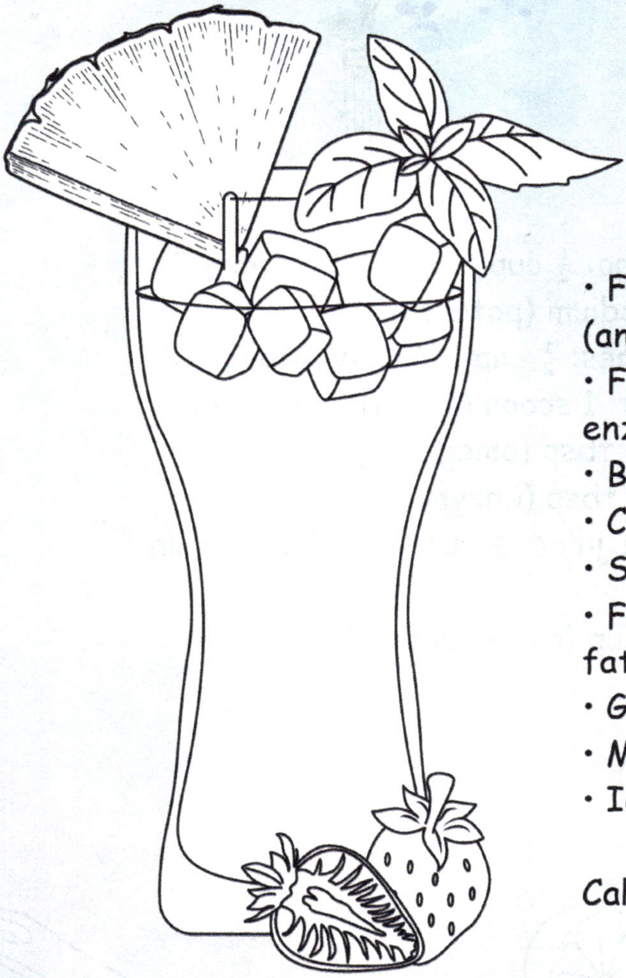

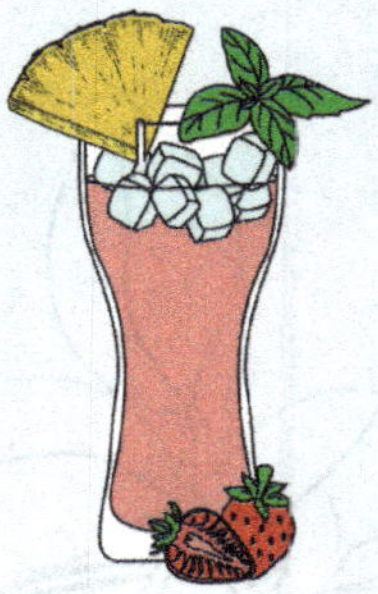

- Frozen strawberries: $\frac{1}{2}$ cup (antioxidants)
- Frozen pineapple: $\frac{1}{2}$ cup (digestive enzymes)
- Banana: $\frac{1}{2}$ medium (potassium)
- Cooked quinoa: 2 tbsp (complete protein)
- Shredded coconut: 1 tbsp (MCTs)
- Full-fat coconut milk: $\frac{3}{4}$ cup (healthy fats)
- Greek yogurt: $\frac{1}{4}$ cup (probiotics)
- Maple syrup: 1 tsp (optional)
- Ice: $\frac{1}{2}$ cup

Calories: 420

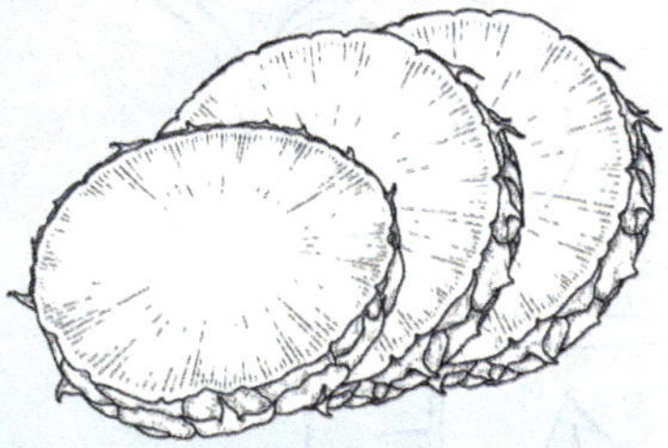

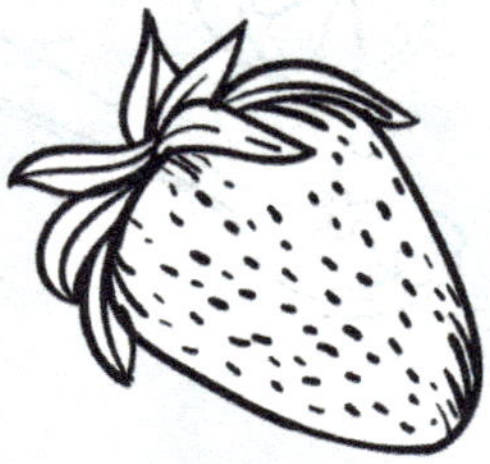

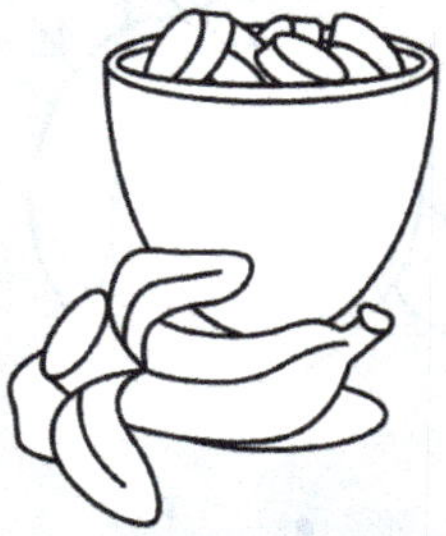

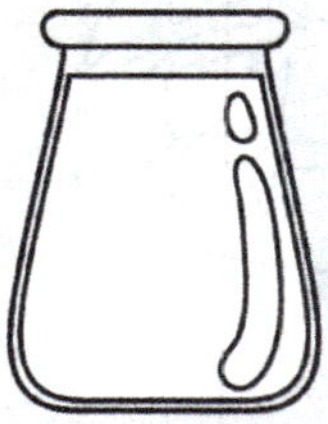

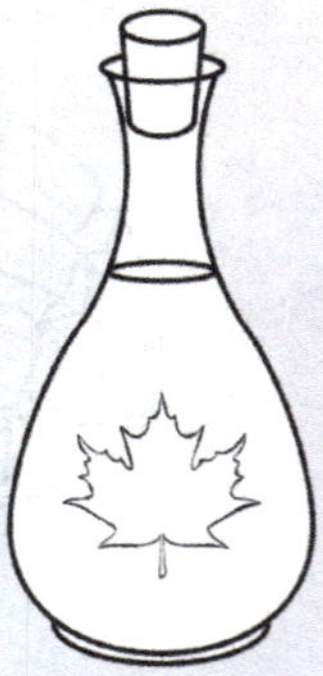

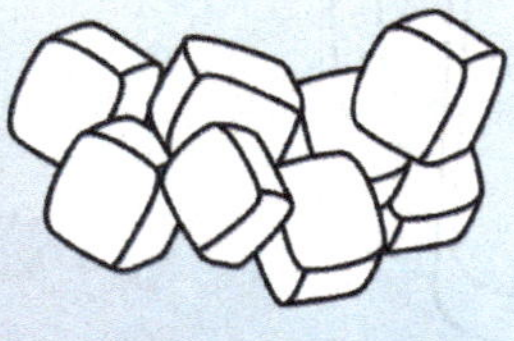

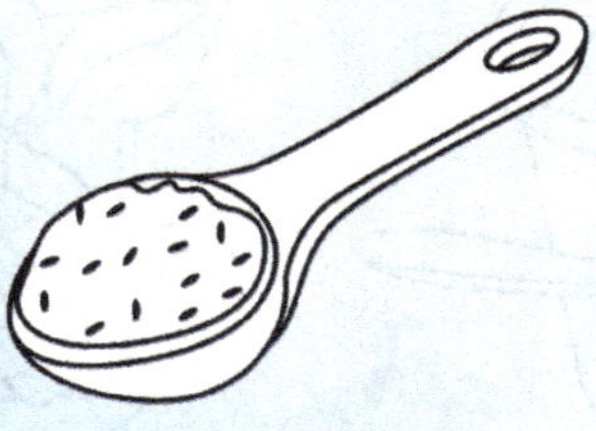

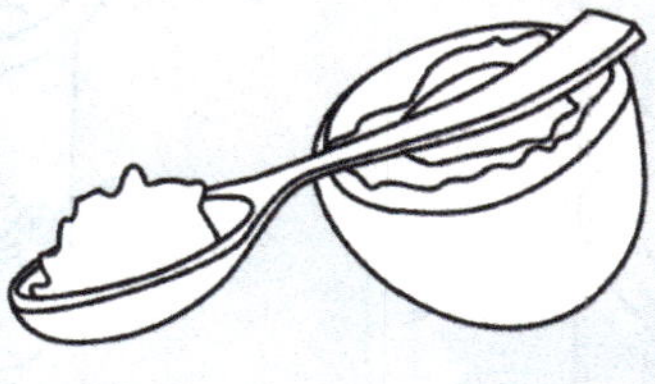

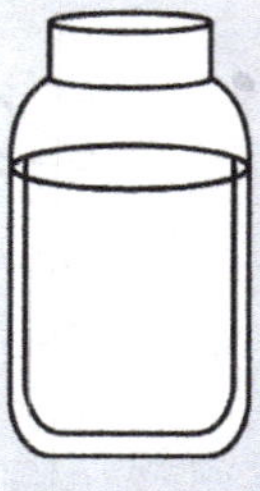

You've built a stable routine. Your stomach works like clockwork, your energy is balanced, and you feel in sync with your body's needs.

Tropical Mango Smoothie Recipe:

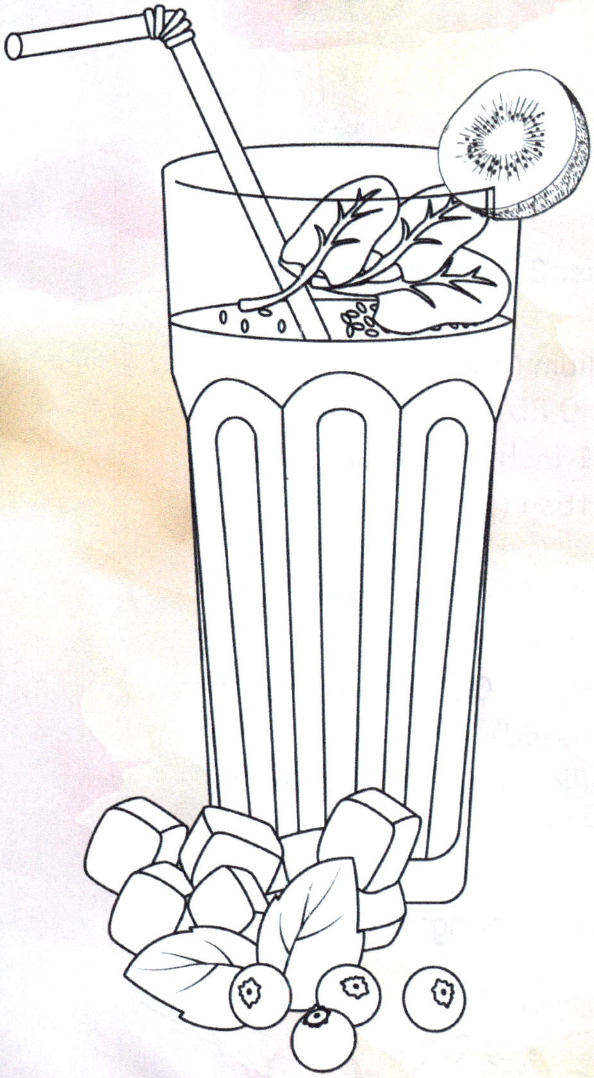

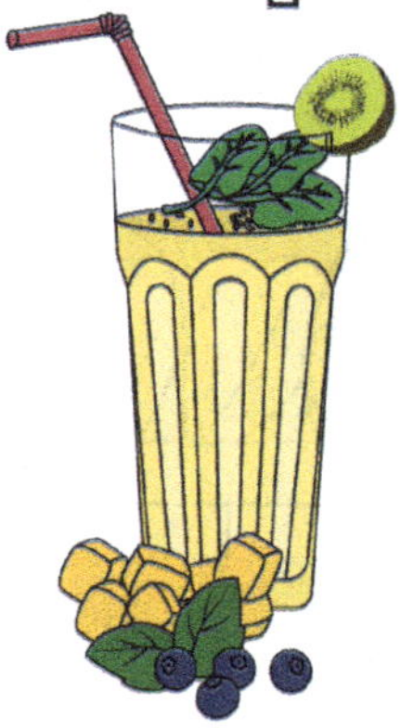

- Frozen mangoes: 2 cups
- Fresh spinach: 2 cups (packed)
- Plant-based yogurt: 1 cup (soy yogurt recommended)
- Ground flax seeds: 2 tbsp
- Plant-based milk: 0.5 cup (unsweetened almond or oat milk)

Optional Toppings:

- Fresh mango chunks
- Kiwi slices
- Blueberries
- Coconut flakes
- Hemp seeds

Calories: ~200

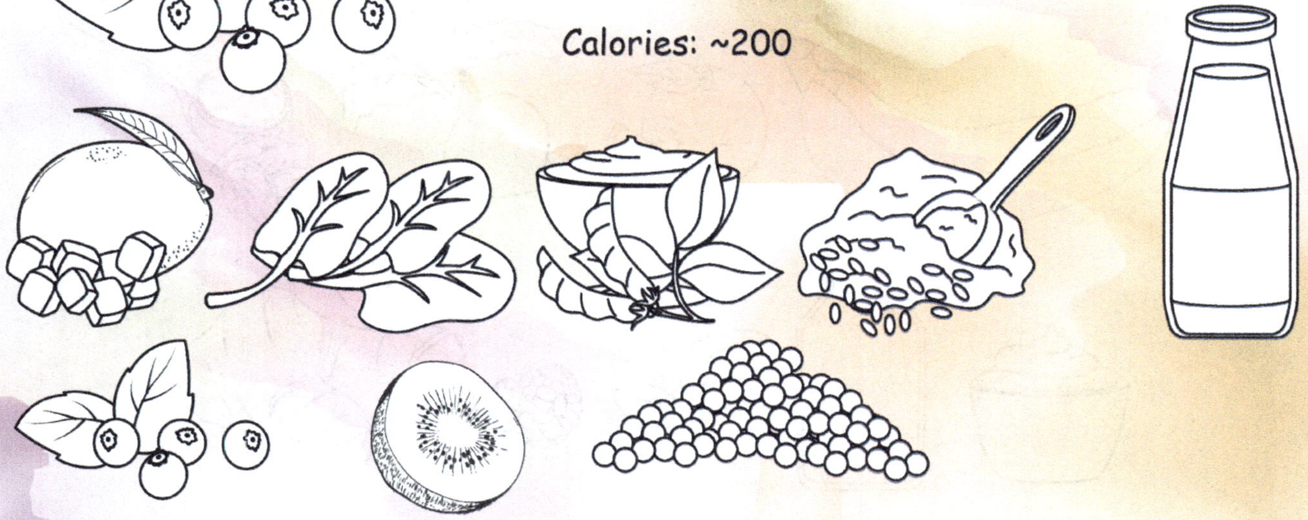

Day 30 – Digestive Reset Complete

Smoothies for breakfast and dinner, high-protein lunch.

Immune-Boosting Green Smoothie:

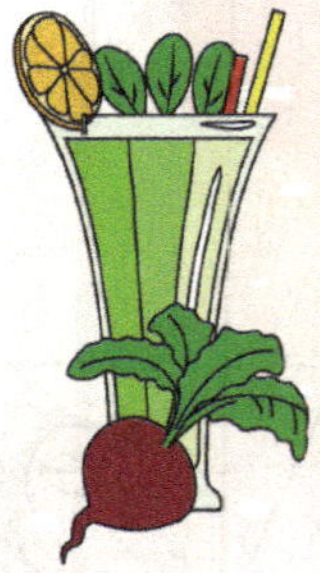

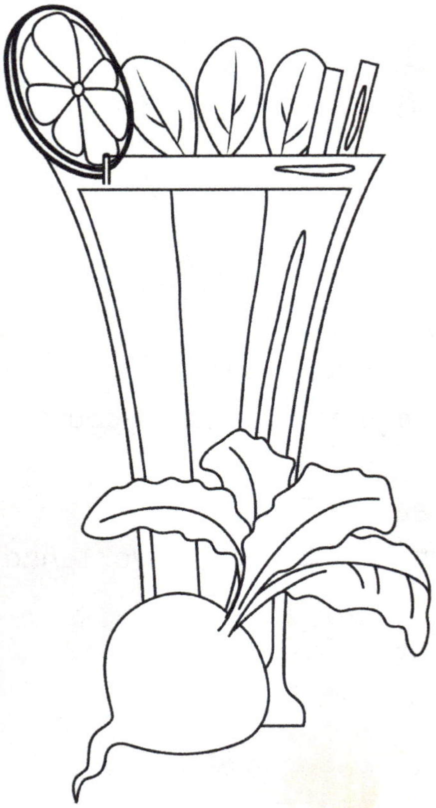

- Frozen bananas: 2 medium (peeled, ~1 cup each)
- Orange: 1 medium (peeled)
- Raw beetroot: 0.25 cup (chopped)
- Fresh ginger: 1-inch chunk (peeled)
- Nut butter: 1 tbsp (peanut or almond butter)
- Spinach: 1 handful (~1 cup packed)
- Frozen raspberries: 0.5 cup
- Plant-based yogurt: 0.25 cup (coconut yogurt recommended)
- Plant-based milk: 1 cup (unsweetened almond or oat milk)

Total calories per serving: ~310 Cal

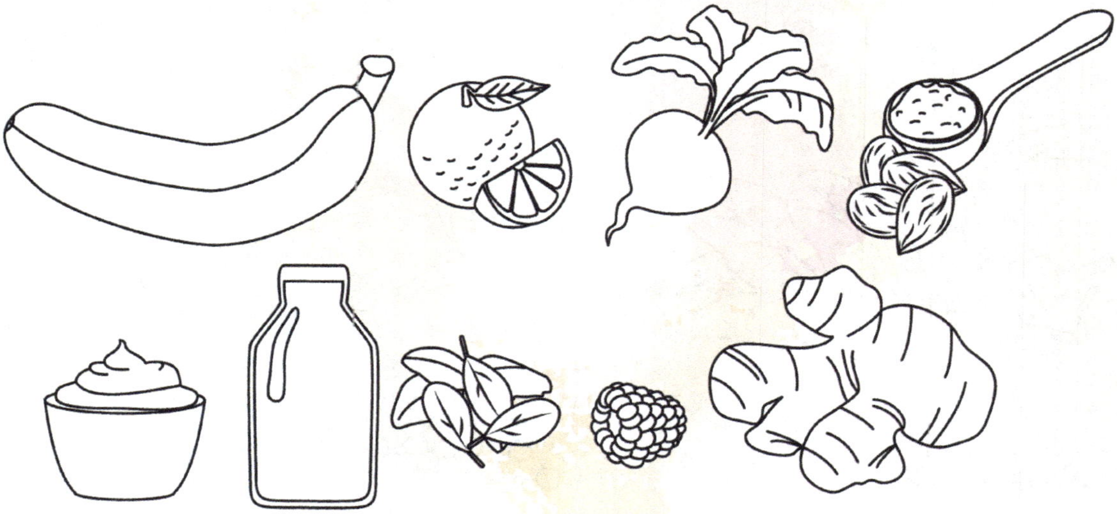

After 30 days, your digestion is lighter, your body is stronger, and your eating habits are cleaner and more intuitive. You've reset not just your stomach — but your entire rhythm.

Introduction to the Sunrise Pink Smoothie:

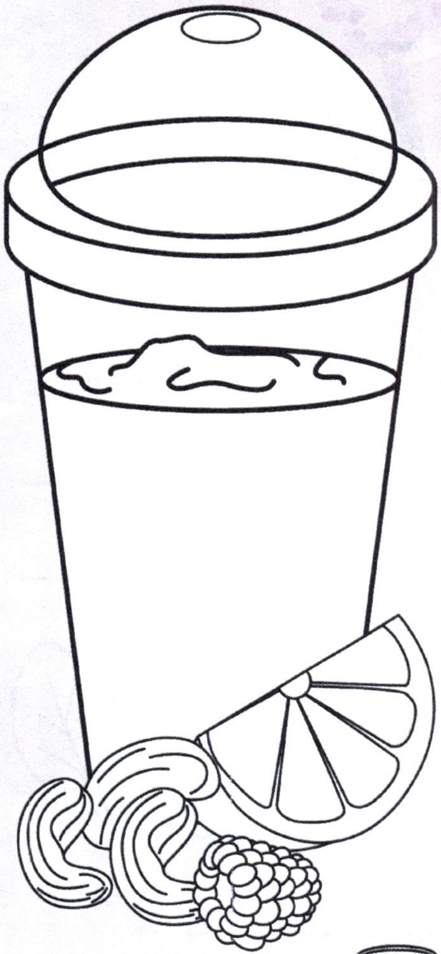

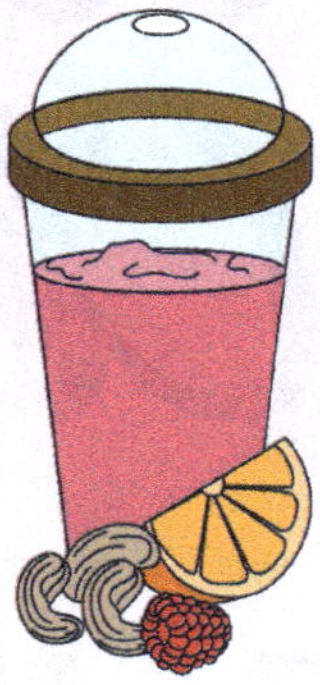

- Orange: 1 medium (peeled)
- Carrot: 1 medium (chopped, ~1/2 cup)
- Small beetroot: 1 (chopped, ~1/2 cup)
- Frozen strawberries: 1 cup
- Frozen zucchini: 0.5 cup
- Frozen raspberries: 1 cup
- Roasted cashews: 0.5 cup
- Plant-based milk: 1.5 cups (coconut milk recommended)

Optional Sweeteners:

- 1 small banana or 2 pitted Medjool dates

Calories: 62 Cal

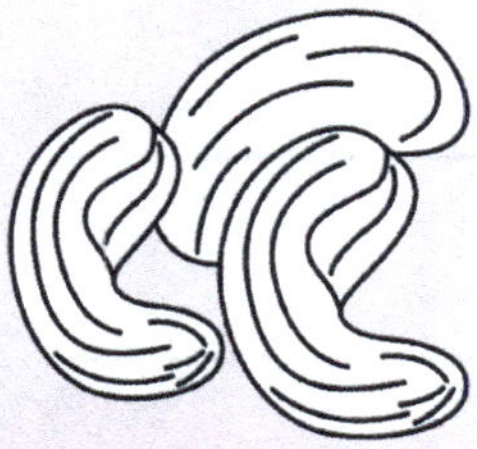

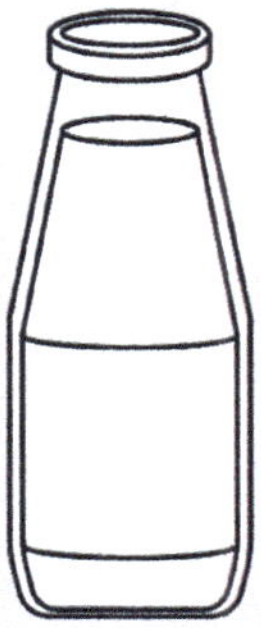

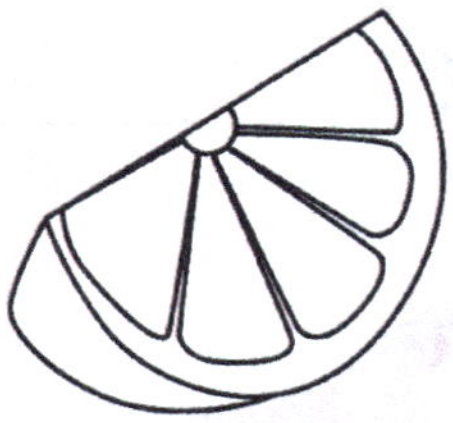

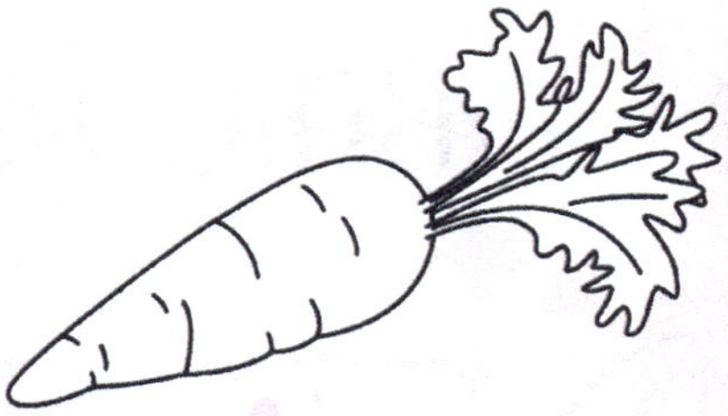

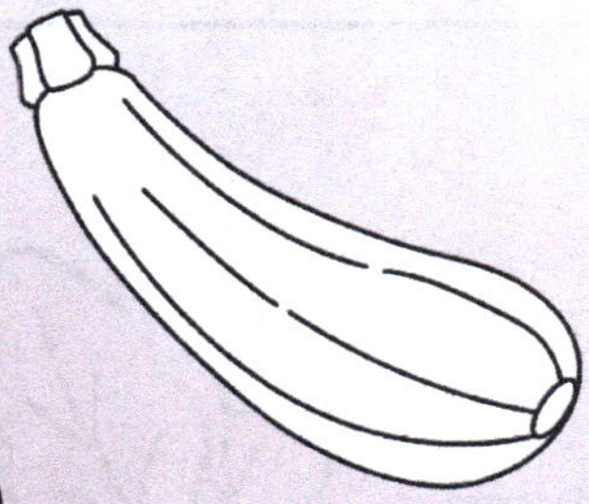

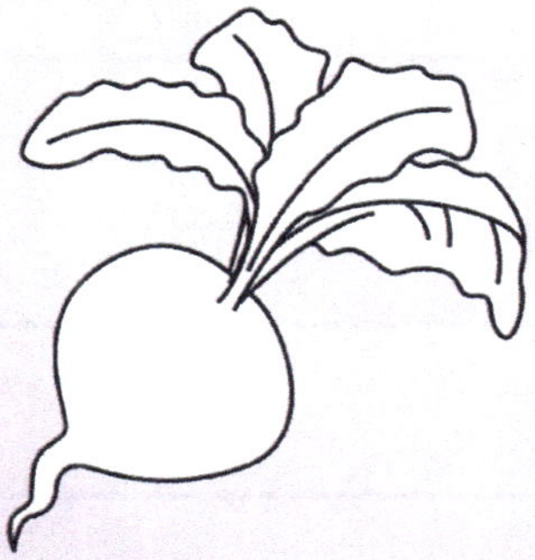

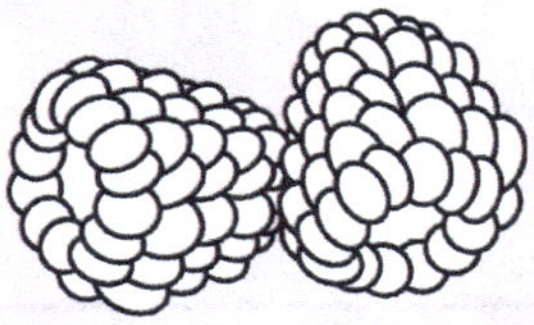

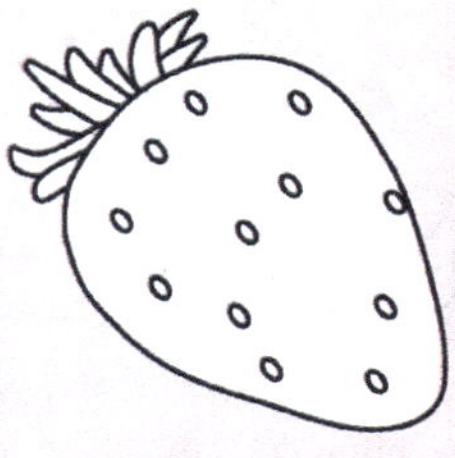

Weekly Wellness Check-In

Weight This Week ______________________

____

____

Favorite Smoothie __________________

____

____

Mood This Week ______________________

____

____

Notes __________________________

____

My Notes & Ideas

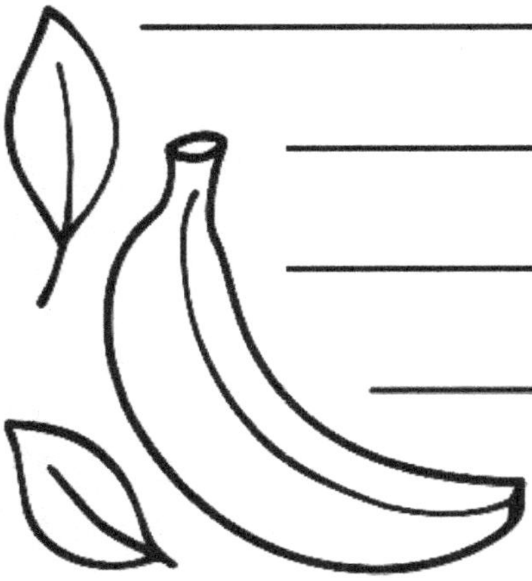

What's Next? – A Glimpse into Book 2

You've completed 30 days. Your digestion is lighter, your body feels refreshed, and your mind is clearer. But this is only the beginning.

Book 2 is not about going back to old habits.
It's about moving forward — with freedom, flexibility, and awareness.
We'll explore how to:

- integrate smoothies into a regular routine without strict rules,
- eat intuitively, but not chaotically,
- structure your week with light "digestive rest" days,
- avoid slipping back into fatigue or stomach discomfort,
- and turn this 30-day reset into a lifestyle, not just a one-time detox.

Book 2 is about long-term balance, energy, and enjoying food without guilt.
Ready to feel light — not just for 30 days, but every day?

Thank you so much for reading this book!

We'd Love to hear from You

Review on Amazon

Scan me

Made in the USA
Monee, IL
02 November 2026

67385563R00044